THE TYPE II DIABETES COOKBOOK

THE TYPE II DIABETES COOKBOOK

Simple and Delicious
Low-Sugar, Low-Fat, and
Low-Cholesterol Recipes

Lois M. Soneral

foreword by
Charles L. Chavez, M.D.

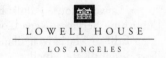

LOWELL HOUSE

LOS ANGELES

CONTEMPORARY BOOKS

CHICAGO

Library of Congress Cataloging-in-Publication Data
Soneral, Lois M.
    The type II diabetes cookbook / Lois M. Soneral ; with a
foreword by Charles L. Chavez.
       p. cm.
    Includes index
    ISBN 1-56565-700-4
    ISBN 1-56565-861-2 (paperback)
    1. Non-insulin-dependent diabetes—Diet therapy—
Recipes.   2. Food exchange lists. I. Title. II. Title:
Type 2 diabetes cookbook.   III. Title: Type two diabetes
cookbook.
RC661.S64 1997
641.5'6314—DC21   97-3177
                                         CIP

Requests for such permissions should be addressed to:
Lowell House
2020 Avenue of the Stars, Suite 300
Los Angeles, CA 90067

Lowell House books can be purchased at special discounts when or-
dered in bulk for premiums and special sales. Contact Department TC
at the address above.

Publisher: Jack Artenstein
Associate Publisher, Lowell House Adult: Bud Sperry
Director of Publishing Services: Rena Copperman
Managing Editor: Maria Magallanes
Text design: Kate Mueller

Manufactured in the United States of America
10 9 8 7 6 5 4 3 2 1

I dedicate this book to my daughters, Ruth Soneral and Janice Soneral Sutula, for their encouragement, support, and love. I hope they will see a world without diabetes.

ACKNOWLEDGMENTS

To my family for all of their support and computer knowledge, for eating the recipes that I modified as well as the new ones I created; for their knowledge of nutrition; and mostly for caring about me, talking with and listening to me.

Special thanks to my daughter, Janice Soneral Sutula, for being there for me to help me get to where I am at now.

To my husband, Carl Soneral, for eating the food I experimented with and for taking me out to eat when an experiment ended up in the garbage disposal.

To my daughter, Ruth Soneral, for making me go to the hospital, although I was in New Mexico and she was in Michigan, but mostly for all the time and effort she contributed to making this book a reality.

To my son-in-law, Ronald Sutula, for giving me an arm to lean on.

To Charles L. Chavez, M.D., without whom I would not be alive and well, nor would I have written this book. He often hosted my "pity parties," talked with me and listened to me. A special thanks for writing the foreword for this book.

To my professional friends who worked diligently with my daughter Janice and me to teach us about diabetes and how to control it.

Special thanks to: LaVerne Hohnstreiter, R.N., C.D.E., of Albuquerque, New Mexico, for encouraging me to get tight control of my diabetes.

To: Beverly J. Spears, R.D., C.D.E., L.D., at the Diabetes Center in Albuquerque, who taught me so much about nutrition and for writing an endorsement for this book.

To: Dottie Gorzynski, B.S.N./R.N., Director of Education at Memorial Medical Center of West Michigan, Mentor of the Diabetes Support Group, who gave me encouragement and wrote an endorsement for this book.

To: Dr. Larry Foster, M.A., D.Min., family therapist, for getting me through the "why me's," and for writing an endorsement for this book.

To: Dr. Alan L. Mast, D.P.M., of the Foot and Ankle Clinic of West Michigan for taking excellent care of my feet and for writing an endorsement for this book.

To: Virginia Valentine, R.N., M.S., C.D.E., of Albuquerque, a thank you for her excerpt about me in her book, *Diabetes Type II & What to Do*.

To: Phyllis Young, Jeanette Petersen, Helen and Arnold Nelson, Lenda Sanches, Carolyn Witter, Harold and Betty Fisher, LeRoy and Helen Petersen, Guy and Nancy Merskin, Patrick Powers, and Ronald Johnson, for all of their help and support.

To my relatives and friends: Thank you for being there for me when I needed you (and even when I didn't), for telling me, "No, you can't have that," for preparing food that I could have when we were invited to your homes, and for knowing what to do when I forgot to eat and went into hypoglycemia. Thank you for all of the prayers that were said in my behalf.

To my diabetes support groups, in Michigan and in New Mexico: for sharing your thoughts and feelings with me.

To my Write People Group: for sharing writing skills.

To the American Diabetes Association: for permission to use their guidelines; to the Memorial Medical Center of West Michigan for permission to use "handouts;" and to Beverly Spears at the Presbyterian Diabetes Center in Albuquerque, for permission to use some materials.

To my pastor, B. Douglas Niemi, and his wife, Patricia, for their emotional and spiritual support, for listening to me and talking with me.

And to God, for giving me the guidance, strength, knowledge, and determination to control my diabetes. He's kept his arm around my shoulder.

CONTENTS

FOREWORD

I met Lois Soneral in an Albuquerque hospital in the spring of 1991. I happened to be on call as the hospital doctor that week. The previous night, my partner had admitted Lois to the intensive care unit. Before I saw her, I reviewed her chart, noted her admission blood sugar, and thought, "This is the highest blood sugar I have ever seen." It was 907. In fact, I have not seen a level that high since. Lois was quite sick, but over the course of a week she improved and was discharged.

Like all new-onset diabetics, she received in-hospital patient education, and arrangements were made for her to have outpatient follow-up, not only by myself but by the Diabetes Center. Lois was initially sent home on subcutaneous insulin and diet modification. Soon it was clear that Lois was not your ordinary new-onset diabetic. She had a long history and strong interest in cooking, and when it was time to get down to day-to-day planning of her meals she easily mastered the task. Along with exercise and regular monitoring of her blood sugar, her diet quickly brought her diabetes under excellent control. Within months, she was able to get off the insulin and did not require any oral hypoglycemic.

Lois had been visiting her daughter in Albuquerque when she got sick. Soon she returned to Michigan, but she spends several months in New Mexico each year, so I get to see her on a regular basis. I have learned that she has been very active in diabetes education in her hometown. She is a member of the diabetes support group there, the American Diabetes Association of Michigan affiliate, as well as the American Diabetes Association. She is also very active in her church as well as other community and crafts organizations. Diabetes has certainly not slowed Lois Soneral. In fact, I think her diabetes and the changes she made as a result have opened her life and given it new meaning.

Over the years, Lois has modified her old recipes and created dozens of new ones. She has shared these with family and friends for years and has now brought them together to share with everyone. The recipes are well thought out. I have used them and recommend them highly.

Charles L. Chavez, M.D.

INTRODUCTION

Diabetes is a genetic disease and a metabolic disorder that affects the way food is converted into energy by the body. I have Type II diabetes; this means my body makes some insulin. In Type I diabetes, which frequently begins in childhood, the pancreas makes no insulin so it has to be injected into the body. The onset of Type II diabetes usually occurs in midlife. The pancreas still produces insulin, but the body's cells cannot make use of the insulin as they should. While most Type I diabetics are of normal weight, Type II diabetics are usually overweight.

March 1, 1991: We were spending the winter in Albuquerque. I had intestinal flu and was unable to keep anything down for four days. I was crawling to the bathroom because I could not stand or walk, but I did not want to go to the hospital. Nevertheless, my family took me to the emergency room at a local hospital, where I was diagnosed with severe dehydration. During a routine examination, my blood glucose reading was taken. It was 907 (normal is between 70 and 120), with a potassium level of 1.4 (normal is 4.0). I had had a physical the previous August and was not diabetic at that time. Other tests were taken, and I was admitted to the intensive care unit. I was still coherent enough to answer questions, and to understand as I was told that I had diabetes. I was placed on insulin injections.

I was hooked up to a lot of wires and tubes, and I remember only a few things from the next three and a half days. I remember that the night shift had pizza brought in and it smelled so good;

I wanted some. This was noted on my chart. The next morning Dr. Charles L. Chavez came in to see me, and said, "Oh, you would like pizza, but will you settle for Jell-O, bouillon, and tea?" I said no, but that is what I got. It ran down my chin, but it tasted good. Later that day I was taken out of ICU and moved to a private room.

Dr. Chavez told me that I had Type II diabetes, and would need to be on insulin. My first reaction was, "What do I do now"? He told me that they would teach me what to do. LaVerne Hohnstreiter, R.N., C.D.E., was going to be my instructor, and other team members from the Diabetes Center in Albuquerque would assist. I had the choice of giving myself injections or having my husband do it. I chose to do it myself. The thought of injecting myself in the stomach for the rest of my life did not appeal to me at all. I knew that I would be a diabetic for the rest of my life, but I vowed I would learn to control it and one day be free of the needle. I was determined to do whatever had to be done to achieve that goal. I was told that I would have to monitor my blood glucose readings; go to classes to learn about diabetes, diet, and nutrition; lose weight; and exercise in order to obtain tight control of my diabetes. The effects on my legs of allergy and skin problems had made it difficult to exercise. I was placed on a strong antibiotic taken internally and also a prescribed cream to be used externally. As my legs began to heal, I began to exercise by walking and climbing stairs.

When I was discharged from the hospital I began going to the Diabetes Center for individual classes, accompanied by my daughter Janice. We learned a lot from the team of professionals there. I also saw Dr. Chavez on a regular basis. I began keeping a journal, writing down everything that I put in my mouth (see Appendix M), my medications (both for my diabetes and my allergies), and my exercise. I was using a Novolin Pen with 70/30 insulin.

I weighed 190 pounds. I wore a women's size 18–20 dress and size 42–44 pants. I resolved to do the best that I could about my weight problem.

After several weeks I was able to return to my home in Michigan. I kept doing the things I had been told to do. I began riding my exercise bike and using stair-steppers, along with walking and stair climbing. This combination has worked very well for me. With monitoring my blood glucose readings, diet, exercise, and close contact with Dr. Chavez and LaVerne Hohnstreiter, I was able to decrease my insulin dosage gradually. When I returned to New Mexico the following winter, I had lost 37 pounds and several inches in girth, and was wearing a size 16 misses. My daughter Janice went with me to see Dr. Chavez. I sat on the examining table and Janice sat on a chair. When he came in, Dr. Chavez said hello, and then said to Janice, "I thought you were bringing your mom in." She said, "I did." He turned to me and said, "Get off that table, I want to look at you." He had not recognized me. He was so pleased with my progress, as were LaVerne and the rest of the team at the Diabetes Center when I went for follow-up instructions. Dr. Chavez said that he had never had a patient accomplish such control over diabetes through weight loss. I had a thorough physical and my team kept decreasing my insulin intake by two units at a time.

I have been off insulin since May 1992 and do not take any oral medication for my diabetes. I monitor my blood glucose readings several times a day, exercise a total of 5½ miles a day, and diligently watch my diet. I still keep a journal, but I no longer write down everything I put in my mouth, unless I am on antibiotics or Prednisone or am traveling. I know what I can and can't have, and although I do not eat what I cannot have, I sometimes eat more of the things that I can have. I watch my intake closely. I have lost 10 more pounds and my weight does not vary by more than 10 pounds. I now wear a size 14, and even have some 12's in my wardrobe.

I am proud of what I have done and of achieving my goal of being free of the needle. And as a wonderful side effect, I'm in a better state of health than I've been in for more than thirty years, even though I'm a diabetic. I have avoided the complications of diabetes and am determined to keep doing so as long as possible. I know that I am an exception and not the rule, but I also know that diabetes is a disease that can be controlled. I am proof that with a lot of determination and effort it can be done.

I wrote this cookbook because diabetics need good, wholesome foods that are not only low in sugar, but also low in fat and cholesterol. We need recipes that are traditional, delicious, and that include easily obtained ingredients—like our mothers used to make. I have found that it is easier to follow my diet when I include some favorite recipes I have modified. I have also included new ones I have developed. Some of these contain a small amount of sugar. Sugar adds more than sweetness, it also adds bulk, which is necessary for a baked product to rise and be light, tender, and delicious.

I am grateful for the excellent sugar substitutes we now have, the availability of fresh fruits and vegetables, and the ease of adding fiber to the diet. Diabetes does not have to be an end to normal living. It can be a beginning to a healthier, happier lifestyle. Following certain guidelines can help you achieve this goal.

1. Monitor your blood glucose levels. Self-monitoring using a blood glucose meter at least twice a day makes your diabetes more manageable.
2. Exercise regularly. Exercise not only burns calories and builds lean tissue (muscle), it increases your basal metabolic rate. For someone suffering from a metabolic disorder like diabetes, this is very important. It means that your body will better convert food into energy all the time—not only when you're exercising, but also when you're at rest.
3. Join a support group. Learn from other members; share your feelings, concerns, problems, and successes with others with this illness. Share coping measures for living with diabetes.
4. Follow your diet. Read labels. Learn to recognize other words for sugar, such as fructose, corn syrup, dextrose, honey, maple syrup, and sorghum. Avoid foods that are high in sugar. If sugar or any of the above is listed as one of the first three ingredients, do not buy the product, as there is a lot of sugar in the product.
5. Learn about your insulin and medications from your doctor. Work with your physician and your other care providers, such as your certified diabetes educator, nutritionist, and dietitian. You are a team.

6. Don't feel overwhelmed by all you need to know. Ask for information and become confident about yourself and your diabetes.

Changes in eating habits are a positive step toward a healthier lifestyle. They make you look and feel better and reduce the risk of a variety of illnesses. A diet that is good for diabetics is good for everyone. You do not have to sacrifice taste or satisfaction. These recipes are so delicious that all of the family can eat the same thing. What's good for you can taste good, too!

EXERCISE IS IMPORTANT FOR DIABETICS

Before becoming a diabetic, I led a sedentary lifestyle. I worked in an office, did crafts, read, and watched TV. I was overweight and I could think of all kinds of excuses not to exercise. I developed a skin infection on my left leg that persisted in spite of antibiotics, and my leg was to be elevated as much as possible. This only gave me more excuses not to exercise.

But when I was told on March 1, 1991, that I have Type II diabetes, the time for all my excuses had ended. Dr. Charles L. Chavez of Albuquerque prescribed a powerful antibiotic, which began to clear up the infection in my leg. He also told me that, because of the diabetes, I had to lose weight, watch my diet, and exercise.

On March 18, 1991, I walked 4 blocks and went up and down 70 stairs. I was exhausted, but I felt good about what I'd done. That was the beginning of my exercise regimen.

By May 1, 1991, when I returned to my home in Michigan,

I was walking 8 blocks and climbing about 100 stairs, up and down. That amount of stair climbing equals about a mile, so my daily total of exercise came to a little over 1.5 miles.

On May 19, 1991, I began riding an exercise bike occasionally. By gradually increasing my exercise, I was averaging 3 miles a day by September 1, 1991. I was losing weight and my insulin intake was being decreased gradually; that kept me motivated to continue.

In March 1992 I added using a stair-stepper to my exercise program. Between the stair-stepper, climbing stairs, walking, and bike riding, I was doing 4 miles a day.

In May 1992 I was taken off insulin. By that time, I was controlling my diabetes with diet and exercise alone. "The team" decided that my goal for the exercise program should be 5.5 miles per day between the combination of walking, riding the exercise bike, climbing stairs, and using the stair-stepper. (I was told that if I was out shopping and hit my 5.5-mile limit, I was *not* to stand in the middle of the parking lot yelling for someone to go get the car and pick me up because I'd just reached my 5.5 miles. I was assured it was OK to exceed my limit by walking to the car.) This combination works well for me.

I set aside enough time after breakfast to put in 3 miles. I keep a journal in which I record my exercise program daily. I exercise even when I have allergy problems or don't feel well, but I do it for shorter periods and more often.

My immediate goal was to get off insulin, which I've achieved, but I have also experienced the following "side effects": I have lost weight; I have tight control of my blood glucose levels; and I am in a better state of health than I've been in for many years—even though I am a diabetic. I continue to be motivated by being able to stay off all medications for diabetes; being able to maintain my weight; feeling great and looking good; and avoiding the complications of diabetes for as long as possible. I will keep doing whatever it takes to keep this up; I've resolved to be the best controlled diabetic I can be.

I know that controlling diabetes is possible if you are motivated and determined to do it. I am proud of what I've done and I know that you can do it, too. Do those exercises that appeal to you and that you can do easily and often. "Cross-train"—do more than one type of exercise, not only so that you exercise different muscles, but also for the psychological advantages of variety. Exercise every day. Do some activity where you are on your feet; it will help avoid complications of diabetes to the feet.

Exercise improves your metabolism and, along with diet, lowers and controls your blood glucose readings, promotes weight loss, makes you look and feel better, makes you feel good about yourself, and helps you avoid complications by taking tight control of your diabetes.

WHY I HAVE INCLUDED SO MANY DESSERTS AND CASSEROLES IN THIS BOOK

When I became diabetic and bought diabetic cookbooks, I often did not find what I was looking for. I began to modify recipes from these cookbooks, as well as family favorite recipes that I had been using for years. I also started to create new recipes as I learned more about nutrition and healthier ways of cooking.

I took these new creations to potlucks, picnics, and parties. I also served them at home to my family and friends. We sometimes voted on a dish to decide if it was "a keeper" or if it needed more work.

People began to ask me for my recipes, which I gladly shared with family and friends. They began encouraging me to write them down. I also shared recipes with my professional friends, who encouraged me to gather them into a book. I did not want to work that hard because I was retired, but that excuse was not a valid one to anyone but me.

I was asked mostly for desserts, casseroles, appetizers, and snacks. People gave this kind of reasoning: "Diabetics cannot have desserts," or "I'll never be able to have pie again." My response was, "Why not?" For this reason this book is "top heavy" with desserts, casseroles, appetizers, and snacks. These are the foods that are not adequately addressed in most other diabetic cookbooks and are clearly what diabetics want. These foods, modified for the needs of diabetics, will make us less inclined to "cheat" on our diets.

APPETIZERS, SNACKS, AND SPREADS

Onion Crisps, Norwegian Style

¾ cup low-fat mayonnaise
1 envelope onion soup mix
8-ounce box Norwegian-style crackers
8 ounces Parmesan cheese, grated
2 teaspoons paprika (or to taste)

Preheat oven to 400°. In a small bowl, mix together the mayonnaise and onion soup mix. Set aside. Remove sheets of the crackers from the package and cut into 1-inch strips. Place on ungreased cookie sheet. Sprinkle with the Parmesan cheese and paprika. Bake at 400° for 2 to 3 minutes, being careful not to let crackers burn. Remove from oven. Spoon on the mayonnaise and onion mix. Allow to cool. Place crackers in a plastic bag and freeze to blend the flavors. Thaw before serving.

YIELD: 150 SMALL CRISPS
SERVING SIZE: 5 CRISPS
EXCHANGES: 1 STARCH/BREAD; 1 FAT

Seasoned Oyster Crackers

❦

I like to use Sunshine Krispy™ crackers for this, as they have no cholesterol.

11-ounce box oyster crackers
0.4-ounce package dry ranch dressing with buttermilk
3 tablespoons gourmet butter-flavor popcorn oil

In a large bowl, combine all the ingredients and mix well. Store in a large plastic or glass container, tightly covered, for up to thirty days. Storing enhances the flavor.

SERVING SIZE: 22 CRACKERS
EXCHANGE: 1 FAT; UP TO 22 CRACKERS IS A FREE FOOD

Italian Pita Squares

2 pitas, about 6 inches in diameter
2 teaspoons "lite" margarine, melted
¼ teaspoon garlic powder
¼ teaspoon oregano or basil
1 teaspoon grated Parmesan cheese

Preheat oven to 350°. Brush pitas with margarine. Sprinkle with garlic powder, oregano, and cheese. Bake 8 to 10 minutes or until lightly browned. Cut each pita into 4 wedges and serve at once.

YIELD: 8 APPETIZERS
SERVING SIZE: ¼ PITA WEDGE
CALORIES: 39
EXCHANGES: ½ STARCH/BREAD

1 G FAT
0 G FIBER
2 G PROTEIN
6 G CARBOHYDRATES

98 MG SODIUM
18 MG POTASSIUM
0 MG CHOLESTEROL

Cereal Party Mix

2 tablespoons margarine
½ teaspoon seasoned salt
2 teaspoons Worcestershire sauce
1 cup rice cereal
1 cup wheat cereal
1 cup thin pretzel sticks (about 90 sticks)
½ cup small cheese crackers, such as Cheez-its™
(about 30 crackers)

Preheat oven to 250°. Melt margarine in a shallow pan. Stir in salt and Worcestershire sauce. Add remaining ingredients. Stir to coat pieces with margarine. Spread mix on a baking sheet and place in 250° oven 45 minutes, stirring every 10 to 15 minutes. Spread on paper toweling to cool. Store in an airtight container.

YIELD: 4 CUPS;
8 SERVINGS
SERVING SIZE: ½ CUP
CALORIES: 100
EXCHANGES: 1 STARCH/
BREAD; ½ FAT

4.1 G FAT
1.1 FIBER
1.8 G PROTEIN
14.6 CARBOHYDRATES

291 MG SODIUM
54.2 MG POTASSIUM
3 MG CHOLESTEROL

Surprise Puffs

❦

8-ounce package refrigerator biscuits
20 cubes cooked chicken or turkey (approximately 6 ounces)
½ cup grated low-fat cheese, such as mozzarella, cheddar,
or any other cheese
½ teaspoon garlic powder
1 teaspoon basil
½ teaspoon onion powder

Preheat oven to 350°. Remove biscuit dough from carton. Cut each biscuit in half and flatten. In the center of each flattened biscuit, place 1 cube of meat, then top with 1 teaspoon cheese. Sprinkle with garlic powder, basil, and onion powder. Seal edges tightly. Arrange seam side down on cookie sheet. Bake at 350° for 10 to 15 minutes or until golden brown.

YIELD: 20 PUFFS	4.4 G FAT	420 MG SODIUM
SERVING SIZE: 2 PUFFS	8.1 G PROTEIN	9.6 MG CHOLESTEROL
CALORIES: 127	13.8 CARBOHYDRATES	

Snack Bites

1 beaten egg

1 tablespoon prepared mustard

1 tablespoon catsup

1 cup whole-wheat bread crumbs

2 tablespoons chopped onion

½ pound ground turkey or chicken

3-ounce can deviled ham

½ cup unsalted cracker crumbs

Preheat oven to 400°. Mix egg, mustard, and catsup. Stir in bread crumbs and onion. Add turkey or chicken and deviled ham. Mix well. Form into 1-inch balls and roll in cracker crumbs. Place on ungreased baking sheet and bake at 400° for 15 minutes.

YIELD: 30 BITES;   3.5 G FAT   36.6 MG CHOLESTEROL
15 SERVINGS   7.4 G PROTEIN
SERVING SIZE: 2 BITES   7.3 MG CARBOHYDRATES
CALORIES: 90
EXCHANGES: ½ STARCH/
BREAD; 1 LEAN MEAT

Popcorn, Southwest Spanish Style

3 tablespoons margarine, melted
3 cups microwave-popped popcorn
¼ teaspoon paprika
⅛ teaspoon garlic powder
⅛ teaspoon red pepper
⅛ teaspoon salt

Drizzle melted margarine over popcorn and stir until well coated. Stir together seasonings. Sprinkle the popcorn with the spice mixture, and stir well again.

YIELD: 2 SERVINGS
SERVING SIZE: 1½ CUPS
EXCHANGES: ½ STARCH/BREAD; ½ FAT

Savory Tuna Spread

✿

7.5-ounce can water-packed tuna

¾ cup low-fat cottage cheese

2 tablespoons chopped green onion

2 teaspoons lemon juice

½ teaspoon black pepper

¼ teaspoon celery powder

¼ cup chopped parsley (optional)

Combine all ingredients. Use a blender if smoother texture is desired.

YIELD: 2 CUPS; 8 SERVINGS   12 G PROTEIN   18 MG CHOLESTEROL
SERVING SIZE: ¼ CUP   1.8 G CARBOHYDRATES
CALORIES: 55

Chicken Spread

1 pound ground chicken

1 small onion, minced

1 teaspoon garlic powder

1 teaspoon basil

½ teaspoon thyme

¼ teaspoon salt

¼ teaspoon black pepper

1 tablespoon apple juice

Sauté the chicken, onion, garlic, basil, and thyme in a medium skillet over medium heat, until browned. Cool. Add salt, pepper, and apple juice. Mix well, using a blender if smoother texture is desired. Cover and chill for several hours. Serve on bread, crackers, or toast.

YIELD: 1½ CUPS; 6 SERVINGS   4 G FAT   294 MG SODIUM
SERVING SIZE: ¼ CUP   12 G PROTEIN
CALORIES: 97   2 G CARBOHYDRATES
EXCHANGES: 1 MEAT

Tuna Sandwich Filling

6-ounce can water-packed tuna

¼ cup chopped celery

1 tablespoon chopped green pepper

1 tablespoon chopped onion

1 tablespoon grated Parmesan or any other cheese

¼ cup plain nonfat yogurt

¼ teaspoon lemon juice

⅛ teaspoon salt

⅛ teaspoon black pepper

Drain the tuna, and flake into a bowl. Add all remaining ingredients and mix well.

YIELD: ¾ CUP; 3 SERVINGS
SERVING SIZE: ¼ CUP
CALORIES: 77

BEVERAGES

Any Color Slush

1 large (8 servings) package sugar-free gelatin, any flavor

2 cups hot water

1 cup cold water

12-ounce can frozen lemonade concentrate

1½ cups unsweetened pineapple juice

48 ounces diet lemon-lime soda

Pour boiling water over the gelatin, stirring until dissolved. Add 1 cup cold water, lemonade concentrate, and pineapple juice. Stir. Freeze until firm. Remove from freezer and pour diet soda over frozen mixture. Stir to form slush. (The mixture may be frozen in 4 small containers and each stirred with a 12-ounce can of diet soda as needed.)

YIELD: 20 SERVINGS   0 G FAT   25 MG SODIUM
SERVING SIZE: ¾ CUP   0 G PROTEIN
CALORIES: 50   14 G CARBOHYDRATES
EXCHANGES: 1 FRUIT

Black Cow Drink

½ cup skim milk

¾ cup diet root beer

¾ cup ice cubes

½ teaspoon vanilla

Place all ingredients in blender and blend until smooth.

YIELD: 2 CUPS   0 G FAT   32 MG SODIUM
SERVING SIZE: 1 CUP   2 G PROTEIN   102 MG POTASSIUM
CALORIES: 21   3 G CARBOHYDRATES   1 MG CHOLESTEROL

So-Easy Fruit Cooler

¾ cup crushed ice (or 6 ice cubes)

1 orange, peeled and cut into chunks

1 banana, peeled and cut into chunks

12-ounce can diet ginger ale

Mix ice, orange, and banana in blender until ice is dissolved. Add ginger ale and mix again. Pour into glasses and serve.

YIELD: 2¼ CUPS   1 G PROTEIN   26 MG SODIUM
SERVING SIZE: ¼ CUP   15 G CARBOHYDRATES
CALORIES: 60

Strawberry Shake

1 cup skim or low-fat (2 percent) milk
¾ cup strawberries (fresh or frozen, unsweetened)
½ cup low-fat frozen vanilla yogurt

Put milk and berries in blender. Blend 10 seconds. Add yogurt and blend until smooth. Serve immediately.

YIELD: 2¼ CUPS;	1.2 FAT	59 MG SODIUM
3 SERVINGS	0.8 FIBER	240 MG POTASSIUM
SERVING SIZE: ¾ CUP	3.9 PROTEIN	4 MG CHOLESTEROL
CALORIES: 75	11.4 G CARBOHYDRATES	

Low-Calorie Eggnog

✻

2 eggs, separated
4 cups low-fat (2 percent) milk
3 packets sugar substitute
1 teaspoon vanilla
½ teaspoon rum flavoring or other flavoring
sprinkle of nutmeg

Combine the egg yolks and milk in a saucepan. Cook over medium heat until the mixture coats a metal spoon. Cool. Beat the egg whites until soft peaks form. Add to the egg custard mixture with the sweetener, vanilla, and rum flavoring. Mix lightly. Cover and chill. Pour into serving cups and sprinkle with nutmeg.

YIELD: 4 CUPS; 8 SERVINGS
SERVING SIZE: ½ CUP
CALORIES: 70
EXCHANGES: 1 MILK; 1 FAT

Raspberry Smoothie

¼ cup unsweetened pineapple juice
½ cup raspberries
1 kiwi fruit, peeled and sliced
3 ice cubes

Reserving a few berries or kiwi slices for garnish, combine all the ingredients in a blender and mix until smooth. Pour into glasses. Garnish with raspberries or kiwi slices.

YIELD: 2 SERVINGS
SERVING SIZE: 3 OUNCES
CALORIES: 50
EXCHANGES: 1 FRUIT

Sober Champagne

½ cup diet ginger ale, chilled
½ cup apple cider, chilled

Mix together and stir well.

YIELD: 1 SERVING
EXCHANGES: 1 FRUIT

Breakfast Shake

½ cup low-calorie citrus punch
½ peeled banana
¼ cup low-fat vanilla yogurt
1 egg
¼ cup low-fat (2 percent) milk

Place all ingredients in a blender and blend until smooth.

YIELD: 1 SERVING
CALORIES: 185
EXCHANGES: 1½ FRUIT; 1 MILK; 1 MEDIUM-FAT MEAT

Strawberry Shake

Any fruit may be used. This makes a delicious, refreshing beverage.

1 cup low-fat (2 percent) milk
½ cup fresh or frozen strawberries
1 packet sugar substitute

Combine all ingredients in a blender and mix until smooth.

YIELD: 1 SERVING
CALORIES: 130
EXCHANGES: ½ FRUIT; 1 FAT

Strawberry Slush

1 pint strawberries, washed and hulled

2 tablespoons lemon juice, preferably fresh

2 tablespoons lime juice, preferably fresh

2 packets sugar substitute

1 cup diet club soda

½ to 1 cup ice cubes

Place strawberries in blender, reserving a few for garnish. Add remaining ingredients. Blend well until smooth and foamy. Garnish with strawberries or fresh lime or lemon slices.

YIELD: 4 CUPS	0 G FAT	5 MG SODIUM
SERVING SIZE: 1 CUP	1 G FIBER	140 MG POTASSIUM
CALORIES: 26	1 G PROTEIN	0 MG CHOLESTEROL
	6 G CARBOHYDRATES	

Cranberry Apple Tea

2 tablespoons sugar-free tea mix
2 cups unsweetened apple juice
2 cups cranberry juice
2 cinnamon sticks
5 whole cloves

In a large saucepan, combine all ingredients. Bring to a boil. Reduce heat and simmer for 8 to 10 minutes. Remove cinnamon stick and cloves from mixture. May be served hot or cold.

YIELD: 4 CUPS
SERVING SIZE: 1 CUP
CALORIES: 100
EXCHANGES: 2 FRUIT

Low-Calorie Cocoa Mix

❦

By the Batch
6½ cups nonfat dry mild powder
¾ cup cocoa powder (unsweetened)
18 packets sugar substitute, or ¾ cup sugar

Mix together. Use ⅓ cup of mixture to 1 cup hot water per serving; stir well.

By the Cup
⅓ cup nonfat dry milk powder
1 packet sugar substitute, or 2 teaspoons sugar
1 tablespoon cocoa powder (unsweetened), or to taste

Mix together. Add 1 cup hot water and stir well.

CALORIES PER CUP: 100 WITH SUGAR SUBSTITUTE; 132 WITH SUGAR
EXCHANGES: 1 SKIM MILK

Fruit and Yogurt Milkshake

2 cups low-fat (2 percent) milk
1 small (4 servings) package sugar-free instant vanilla pudding
1 cup plain low-fat yogurt
1 cup crushed ice
1 cup strawberries, or 1 medium peach, peeled and sliced;
or 1 medium orange, peeled and sliced

Combine all ingredients in a blender, in order given. Blend 1 minute at high speed.

YIELD: 4 CUPS; 8 SERVINGS   0.3 G FAT   1.5 MG CHOLESTEROL
SERVING SIZE: ½ CUP
CALORIES: 99

Breads, Rolls, and Muffins

Aebleskiver
(Small Danish Pancake Balls)

Aebleskiver recipes come from both sides of my family, and I have had to modify them for my diabetic diet. My ancestors came from Denmark and this was a favorite there and also in their new homes in America. My mother made it often for Sunday evening suppers when we were having guests. She would add pieces of apple or other fruit when the batter was poured into the cups. One day when I was seven or eight years old, I put peanut butter into a whole pan full of them. I had intended to eat them all myself, but somehow they got on the table and I got only two of them. My dad (who didn't like peanut butter very well) asked, "What is this?" I had to confess what I had done. They laughed, but others liked them, so we prepared aebleskiver with peanut butter occasionally. They were served with powdered sugar, maple syrup, jelly, jam, and fruit topping. We often served these at our church's youth fellowship meetings, where they were enjoyed by all, and we still have aebleskiver breakfasts at our church occasionally. To prepare them you need an aebleskiver pan or monk's pan, which is similar to a pancake griddle with cuplike indentations.

4 large eggs, separated

2 cups flour

1 tablespoon sugar

4 teaspoons baking powder

½ teaspoon baking soda

½ teaspoon salt

2 cups buttermilk

2 tablespoons cooking cooking oil

Separate egg yolks and whites; beat egg whites until soft peaks form. Mix dry ingredients. Add to beaten egg yolks, alternately with the buttermilk. Fold in the beaten egg whites. Coat pan with oil. Pour batter into cups in pan. Cook on stovetop until browned. Using a knitting needle or a fork, turn as they start to brown. Serve with syrup, jam, jelly, or a fruit topping of your choice. (I like mine with apples or peanut butter.)

YIELD: APPROXIMATELY 30
SERVING SIZE: 3 PANCAKE
BALLS
CALORIES: 100

4 G FAT
2 G PROTEIN
17 G CARBOHYDRATES

200 MG SODIUM

Appelsin (Danish Orange Bread)

❦

This is a very old family favorite recipe that I have modified to use in my diabetic diet. Food is an important part of my family's heritage. This recipe comes from both sides of my family. We would always have it at Christmas, because oranges were only available during the winter in our area. Now that oranges are always available, I make it more often. It is still a favorite Christmas bread, very different from such breads as banana nut or zucchini. It is definitely orange. I make several loaves early in December and put them in the freezer, and often give them as gifts.

3 cups flour

¼ cup sugar

*sugar substitute equivalent to ½ cup sugar,
preferably acesulfame K*

4 teaspoons baking powder

½ teaspoon salt

1 egg

1¼ cups low-fat (2 percent) milk

¼ cup unsweetened orange juice

1 tablespoon grated orange peel

3 tablespoons melted shortening

¾ cup chopped walnuts

Preheat oven to 350°. Sift dry ingredients together. Add egg, milk, orange juice, orange peel, and shortening and mix until well blended. Add chopped nuts and fold into the mixture. Pour into greased 9-by-5-inch loaf pan and let stand for 15 minutes. Bake at 350° for 1 hour or until tester comes out clean.

YIELD: 10 SLICES
SERVING SIZE: 1 SLICE
CALORIES: 100
EXCHANGE: 1 FRUIT; 1 STARCH/BREAD; 1 FAT

Apple Bread

❦

¼ cup raisins

1 egg

2 tablespoons vegetable oil

½ cup white flour

½ cup whole-wheat flour

1 teaspoon baking powder

¼ teaspoon baking soda

1 teaspoon cinnamon

¼ teaspoon salt

¼ cup unsweetened apple juice

2 apples, preferably Ida red or Cortland, peeled and chopped

Preheat oven to 350°. Soak raisins in hot water about 5 minutes to soften. Drain and set aside raisins. Beat egg with vegetable oil. In a separate bowl, mix flours, baking powder, baking soda, cinnamon, and salt. Add a small amount of flour mixture to oil and egg mixture and stir just enough to moisten. Add apple juice and remaining flour and blend well. Add apples and raisins. Bake in a 9-by-5-inch greased loaf pan at 350° for 45 to 50 minutes or until tester comes out clean. Delicious served warm.

YIELD: 10 SLICES   3.6 G FAT   116 MG SODIUM
SERVING SIZE: 1 SLICE   2 G PROTEIN   27.9 MG CHOLESTEROL
CALORIES: 100   15 G CARBOHYDRATES

Banana Bread

2 bananas

2 eggs

½ cup shortening

10 dates, chopped

1¾ cups flour

2 teaspoons baking powder

1 teaspoon baking soda

1 teaspoon cinnamon

½ teaspoon salt

¼ cup chopped walnuts

Preheat oven to 325°. Mash bananas, add eggs and beat well. Cream shortening and stir into banana mixture; add dates. In a separate bowl mix together flour, baking powder, baking soda, cinnamon, salt, and nuts. Stir into creamed mixture, just enough to moisten. (Do not beat.) Bake in a greased 9-by-5-inch loaf pan at 325° for 45 minutes to 1 hour. Serve slightly warm.

YIELD: 12 SLICES   12.2 FAT   227.9 MG SODIUM
SERVING SIZE: 1 SLICE   3.6 G PROTEIN   46 MG CHOLESTEROL
CALORIES: 222   24.5 G CARBOHYDRATES
EXCHANGES: 1 FRUIT;
1 STARCH/BREAD; 2½ FAT

Banana Nut Bread

❦

¼ cup "lite" margarine

½ cup sugar (up to ¼ cup sugar substitute may be used,
preferably acesulfame K))

1 egg

1 teaspoon vanilla extract

1 cup bran cereal

1½ cups flour

2 teaspoons baking powder

½ teaspoon baking soda

½ teaspoon salt

1½ cups mashed bananas

½ cup chopped walnuts

nonstick vegetable spray

Preheat oven to 350°. Cream together margarine and sugar. Add egg and vanilla and beat well. Add uncooked oat bran cereal. Stir together dry ingredients. Add to batter alternately with bananas, mixing well after each addition. Stir in nuts. Turn into 9-by-5-inch loaf pan coated with nonstick vegetable spray. Bake at 350° 55 to 60 minutes or until tester comes out clean. Remove from pan and cool on a rack.

YIELD: 24 SLICES,   6 G FAT   104 MG SODIUM
3/8 INCH THICK   3 G PROTEIN
SERVING SIZE: 1 SLICE   19 G CARBOHYDRATES
CALORIES: 142
EXCHANGES: 1 STARCH/
BREAD; 1 FRUIT

Banana Apple Muffins

❦

1 large ripe banana, mashed

1⅔ cups skim milk

1 teaspoon peanut or safflower oil, plus extra for coating muffin cups

1 teaspoon vanilla extract

½ cup chopped apples, preferably Ida red or Cortland

¼ cup raisins

2½ cups oat bran

1 tablespoon baking powder

¾ teaspoon baking soda

1 teaspoon cinnamon

Lightly oil 12 muffin cups and dust with a little of the oat bran. Preheat oven to 400°. Mix together banana, milk, oil, vanilla, apples, and raisins in a large bowl. Combine remaining dry ingredients in a separate bowl. Add banana mixture and mix lightly. Fill muffin cups half full with batter. Bake for 25 minutes or until lightly browned. Cool 5 minutes. Serve hot, or turn out on wire rack to cool.

YIELD: 12 MUFFINS
SERVING SIZE: 1 MUFFIN
CALORIES: 165
EXCHANGES: 1½ FRUIT; 1 STARCH/BREAD; 1 FAT

Blueberry Muffins

1⅓ cups flour

⅓ cup sugar or equivalent sugar substitute, preferably acesulfame K

2½ teaspoons baking powder

½ teaspoon salt

1 cup blueberries, fresh or unthawed frozen

¾ cup low-fat (2 percent) milk

1 egg

⅓ cup melted margarine

Preheat oven to 400°. In a large bowl, combine flour, sugar, baking powder, and salt. Stir in blueberries. Add milk, egg, and margarine. Mix until dry ingredients are moistened. The batter will be lumpy. Fill muffin cups half full with batter. Bake at 400° for 25 minutes. Serve warm.

YIELD: 12 MUFFINS
SERVING SIZE: 1 MUFFIN
CALORIES: 150

6.2 G FAT
20.8 G CARBOHYDRATES

Sugar-Free Cinnamon Apple Muffins

✳

oil for coating muffin cups
⅔ cup oat bran
1 cup oat flour
1 tablespoon baking powder
1 teaspoon cinnamon
¾ cup skim or low-fat (2 percent) milk
¾ cup finely chopped apples, preferably
Ida red or Cortland, or unsweetened applesauce
⅔ cup raisins
2 egg whites, stiffly beaten

Oil muffin cups and dust with a little of the oat bran. Preheat oven to 350°. In a large bowl, mix dry ingredients. Add milk and apples and mix, leaving batter a little lumpy. Fold in raisins, then the egg whites. (May also be mixed in a food processor.) Fill muffin cups half full with batter. Bake at 350° for 25 minutes or until lightly browned.

YIELD: 12 MUFFINS
SERVING SIZE: 1 MUFFIN
CALORIES: 110
EXCHANGES: 1 FRUIT; 1 STARCH/BREAD; 1 FAT

Peanut Butter Bread

❧

2 cups flour
4 teaspoons baking powder
⅔ cup natural peanut butter
¼ cup unsweetened apple juice concentrate, thawed
1¼ cups low-fat (2 percent) milk

Preheat oven to 350°. Mix flour and baking powder together in a large bowl. In a separate bowl, mix peanut butter and apple juice concentrate. In a saucepan, heat the milk until lukewarm. Add the peanut butter mixture to the milk and blend well. Combine the wet and dry ingredients and beat thoroughly. Pour into a greased 9-by-5-inch loaf pan. Bake at 350° for 45 to 50 minutes, until tester comes out clean. Cool before slicing.

YIELD: 10 SLICES
SERVING SIZE: 1 SLICE
CALORIES: 120
EXCHANGES: 1 STARCH/BREAD; 1 HIGH-FAT MEAT

Zucchini Bread

3 cups flour

2 teaspoons cinnamon

1 teaspoon baking soda

¼ teaspoon baking powder

2 cups grated zucchini

3 eggs

1 cup unsweetened apple juice concentrate, thawed

½ cup cooking oil

3 teaspoons vanilla

1 cup chopped walnuts

Preheat oven to 350°. Mix together the dry ingredients. In a separate bowl, mix the moist ingredients. Blend the two mixtures together. Add the chopped walnuts. Pour into 2 greased 9-by-5-inch loaf pans. Bake a 350° for 1 hour, or until tester inserted in center comes out clean. (*Note:* This bread freezes very well.)

YIELD: 24 SLICES
SERVING SIZE: 1 SLICE
CALORIES: 161
EXCHANGES: 1 STARCH/
BREAD; 2 FAT;
½ VEGETABLE

9 G FAT
3 G PROTEIN
17 G CARBOHYDRATES

47 MG SODIUM
35 MG CHOLESTEROL

SOUPS

Tortilla Soup

❧

6 corn tortillas

1 medium onion, chopped

3 cloves garlic, minced

1 tablespoon olive oil

2 tablespoons chili powder

1 teaspoon oregano

28-ounce can concentrated crushed tomatoes

10-ounce can low-fat chicken broth, plus 1 can water

1 green pepper, diced

1 cup fresh or frozen corn kernels

salt and pepper to taste

1. About 15 minutes before you plan to serve soup, heat tortillas in a 325° oven until crisp.
2. In a soup pot, sauté onion and garlic in oil until soft. Stir in chili powder and oregano. Stir in tomatoes, chicken broth, and water. Bring to a boil and simmer for a few minutes. Add corn and green pepper. Add salt and pepper to taste.

3. For each serving, break a tortilla into small pieces and place at bottom of a soup bowl. Ladle soup over the tortilla and serve.

YIELD: 6 SERVINGS
CALORIES: 155

3.5 G FAT (21% CALORIES FROM FAT)
389 MG SODIUM
0 MG CHOLESTEROL

Cucumber Buttermilk Soup

2 cups buttermilk
½ cup seeded, shredded cucumber
1 tablespoon snipped parsley
1 tablespoon sliced green onion
½ teaspoon dried dillweed
½ teaspoon instant chicken bouillon granules
dash black pepper

Combine all ingredients. Place in covered container and chill at least 3 hours, up to 24 hours. This soup should be served icy cold.

YIELD: 2 CUPS
SERVING SIZE: 1 CUP
CALORIES: 65
EXCHANGES: 1 MILK; ¼ VEGETABLE

Broccoli Cheese Soup

1 cup chopped fresh or frozen broccoli
3 cups water
2 yellow onions, thinly sliced
1½ tablespoons flour
½ teaspoon salt
2 cups low-fat (2 percent) milk
½ cup low-fat grated cheddar cheese

Cook the broccoli in the water with the onions, until the broccoli is tender. Cool and puree in a blender. Return the puree to the pan. Combine the flour, salt, and milk in a bowl. Stir the flour mixture into the pureed broccoli and simmer over medium heat until thickened, about 15 minutes. Add the cheese and stir until melted. Remove from the heat and serve.

YIELD: 4 SERVINGS   12 G FAT   464 MG SODIUM
SERVING SIZE: 1 CUP   11 G PROTEIN
CALORIES: 241

Swedish Fruit Soup

✤

Our Swedish friends and families served this at Christmastime and other special occasions. It can be served either hot or cold with a spoonful of yogurt. I like it hot at a meal.

3 cups mixed dried fruit (apricots, peaches, pears, apples)
½ cup pitted prunes
½ cup raisins
6 cups water
2 tablespoons honey
¼ teaspoon ground mace
1 cinnamon stick (3 inches long)
1 cup yogurt

In a saucepan, combine all the ingredients except the yogurt. Bring to a boil, cover, and simmer for 1 hour or until fruit is tender. Remove the cinnamon stick. Serve soup hot or cold with a spoonful of yogurt.

YIELD: 8 CUPS; 16 SERVINGS
SERVING SIZE: ½ CUP
CALORIES: 109
EXCHANGES: 1 FRUIT

French Onion Soup

1½ cups thinly sliced onions
2 tablespoons "lite" margarine or oil
6 cups beef broth
1½ teaspoons freshly ground black pepper (or to taste)
6 slices French bread, toasted
6 slices low-fat mozzarella cheese, grated or shredded

Sauté onions in margarine or oil until transparent and thoroughly cooked. Add broth and black pepper. Simmer 30 minutes. Divide into 6 ovenproof casseroles or bowls. Top each with a slice of toasted French bread and sprinkle with mozzarella. Place in a 350° oven until cheese is melted. Serve immediately.

YIELD: APPROX. 1½ QUARTS;	8 G FAT	325 MG SODIUM
6 SERVINGS	8 G PROTEIN	
SERVING SIZE: 1 CUP	22 G CARBOHYDRATES	
CALORIES: 165		

SALADS AND DRESSINGS

Apple Orange Pinwheel Salad

2 apples, preferably red or golden delicious, Ida red, or Cortland

2 oranges

8 leaves of lettuce

Core and slice apples. Peel and slice oranges. Arrange lettuce with apple and orange "wheels" alternately on top.

YIELD: 8 SERVINGS   0.3 G FAT   2 MG SODIUM

CALORIES: 64   2.3 G FIBER   216.5 MG POTASSIUM

     0.9 G PROTEIN   0 MG CHOLESTEROL

     16.3 G CARBOHYDRATES

Black Cherry Salad

⚜

8-ounce package nonfat cream cheese
14-ounce can black sweet cherries, drained; reserve juice
¼ cup cold water
1 small (4 servings) package sugar-free cherry gelatin
1 cup boiling water
8 ounces nonfat whipped topping

Place cream cheese in a bowl. Add 2 tablespoons of the reserved cherry juice and ¼ cup cold water. Beat well with an electric mixer. Mix gelatin with boiling water and add to cream cheese mixture; blend well. Fold in drained cherries and whipped topping; blend well. Pour into 9-by-13-inch pan and refrigerate several hours.

YIELD: 9 SERVINGS
SERVING SIZE: 1 3-BY-4-INCH SQUARE
CALORIES: 105

0 G FAT
2 G FIBER
20 G CARBOHYDRATES

Molded Apple Salad

❦

1 small (4 servings) package sugar-free strawberry gelatin
¾ cup boiling water
⅓ unsweetened apple juice
ice cubes
1 medium unpeeled apple, chopped (about 1¼ cups)
½ cup chopped celery

Dissolve gelatin in boiling water. Combine apple juice and ice cubes to make 1¼ cups liquid. Add to gelatin and stir until slightly thickened. Remove any unmelted ice. Add apples and celery. Chill until set, about 2 to 2½ hours.

YIELD: 5 SERVINGS	0 G FAT	16 MG SODIUM
SERVING SIZE: ½ CUP	8 G CARBOHYDRATES	
CALORIES: 35		

Waldorf Salad

4 teaspoons low-fat mayonnaise
2 teaspoons unsweetened pineapple juice
3 small red apples
½ cup diced celery
¼ cup chopped walnuts

Mix mayonnaise with pineapple juice. Dice unpeeled apples. Mix with celery and nuts. Fold in dressing.

YIELD: 4 SERVINGS	8.9 G FAT	41 MG SODIUM
SERVING SIZE: ¾ CUP	2.3 G FIBER	179.3 MG POTASSIUM
CALORIES: 134	1.4 G PROTEIN	3 MG CHOLESTEROL
	14.5 G CARBOHYDRATES	

Strawberry Salad

❦

1 large (8 servings) package sugar-free strawberry gelatin
2 cups boiling water
10-ounce package frozen strawberries, no sugar added
16-ounce can crushed pineapple in its own juice
½ pint "lite" sour cream

Dissolve gelatin in boiling water. Add strawberries and pineapple, include juice. Fill a ring mold with half the mixture and chill for 30 minutes. Add layer of sour cream. Pour the remaining gelatin mixture on top. Chill until firm.

YIELD: 8 SERVINGS
SERVING SIZE: 4 OUNCES
CALORIES: 100
EXCHANGES: 2 FRUIT; ½ FAT

Mandarin Orange Mold

❦

2 envelopes unflavored gelatin

1½ cups boiling water

6-ounce can frozen unsweetened orange juice concentrate

¾ cup cold water

15-ounce can mandarin oranges, drained

Dissolve gelatin in boiling water. Add frozen juice concentrate and cold water. Mix well. Place orange segments in a mold and fill with gelatin mixture. Refrigerate. When almost set, stir to distribute orange segments. Chill well to set gelatin firmly.

YIELD: 4 CUPS; 8 SERVINGS 0.1 G FAT   3.7 MG SODIUM
SERVING SIZE: ½ CUP   0.3 G FIBER   247 MG POTASSIUM
CALORIES 56   2.0 G PROTEIN   0 MG CHOLESTEROL
EXCHANGES: 1 FRUIT   12.4 CARBOHYDRATES
KEY SOURCE NUTRIENT: 46 MG ASCORBIC ACID

Piña Colada Salad

11-ounce can mandarin oranges, drained; reserve juice

8-ounce can pineapple chunks in own juice, drained; reserve juice

1 banana, sliced and sprinkled with 1 teaspoon lemon juice

1 envelope nonfat whipped topping mix;
or an 8-ounce tub of nonfat whipped topping

½ teaspoon vanilla extract

½ teaspoon rum extract

2 tablespoons toasted coconut flakes

Combine oranges, pineapple, and banana in a mixing bowl. Whip topping with ½ cup fruit juices (use all the pineapple juice and enough liquid from mandarin oranges to make ½ cup total). Whip in vanilla and rum extracts. Fold into fruit mixture; sprinkle with coconut. Chill several hours.

YIELD: 4 SERVINGS
SERVING SIZE: ¾ CUP
CALORIES: 174
EXCHANGES: 2 FRUIT;
1 FAT

5 G FAT
3 G FIBER
1 G PROTEIN
34 G CARBOHYDRATES

13 MG SODIUM
326 MG POTASSIUM
0 MG CHOLESTEROL

Lime Gelatin Salad

1 large (8 servings) package sugar-free lime gelatin
1 cup boiling water
1 cup low-fat cottage cheese
1 cup low-fat mayonnaise, such as Kraft Miracle Whip™
1 cup low-fat (2 percent) milk
16-ounce can crushed pineapple in its own juice

Mix gelatin with boiling water and mix well. Mix cottage cheese and mayonnaise with milk and blend well. Add pineapple and juice; pour into a mold.

YIELD: 8 SERVINGS
SERVING SIZE: ½ CUP
CALORIES: 110
EXCHANGE: 1 FRUIT; 2 FAT

Fruited Chicken Salad

2 cups diced cooked chicken

1 cup halved seedless grapes

2 tablespoons slivered almonds

¼ cup "lite" sour cream

1 tablespoon low-fat mayonnaise

1 cup chopped celery

½ cup canned unsweetened crushed pineapple,
include ½ cup of the juice

½ teaspoon salt (optional)

lettuce

Combine all ingredients and mix well. Chill. Serve on lettuce.

YIELD: 4 SERVINGS	8.3 G FAT	448.4 MG SODIUM
SERVING SIZE: 1 CUP	6.2 G FIBER	905.5 MG POTASSIUM
CALORIES: 245	19.2 G PROTEIN	52 MG CHOLESTEROL
	24.1 G CARBOHYDRATES	

Corned Beef Salad

❦

2 beef bouillon cubes

1 cup hot water

1 cup low-fat mayonnaise, such as Kraft Miracle Whip™

1 large (8 servings) package sugar-free lemon gelatin

1 cup diced celery

3 tablespoons grated onion

3 tablespoons diced green pepper

3 hard-boiled eggs, diced

12-ounce can corned beef, chilled; cut and cubed
(it is easier to cut if chilled)

Mix bouillon cubes in hot water. Add mayonnaise and beat until well mixed. Prepare gelatin in a 9-by-13-inch pan, and refrigerate until you're ready to add the remaining ingredients. Mix celery, onion, green pepper, hard-boiled eggs, and cubed corned beef in a bowl. Pour mixture into the 9-by-13-inch pan. Mix with gelatin and chill until set.

YIELD: 10 SERVINGS
SERVING SIZE: 1 3-BY-3½-INCH PIECE
CALORIES: 180
EXCHANGES: 2 MEDIUM-FAT MEAT; 1 VEGETABLE; 1 FAT

Chicken Salad

1 cup finely chopped cooked chicken
½ cup finely chopped celery
½ cup low-fat mayonnaise, such as Kraft Miracle Whip™
2 tablespoons low-fat Italian dressing
2 onions, finely chopped
1 teaspoon prepared mustard
salt and pepper to taste
dash of paprika

Mix all the ingredients except the paprika. Refrigerate. (May be made a day ahead.) Sprinkle with paprika and serve.

YIELD: 4 SERVINGS
SERVING SIZE: ½ CUP
CALORIES: 240
EXCHANGE: 1 MEAT; 1 FAT

Hot Tuna Salad

❦

This dish began as an experiment. My family likes tunafish salad, but it is always served cold. Why couldn't it be served hot? I decided to work on it. It was a disaster and promptly went into the garbage disposal; my husband took me out to eat. But, being stubborn, I persisted and after several attempts, finally got it right! It has a different taste and texture from cold tuna salads, and our friends like it.

2 hard-boiled eggs

10¾-ounce can cream of chicken or cream of mushroom soup, condensed

6-ounce can water-packed tuna

2 ribs celery

½ cup frozen peas

¼ cup chopped onion

¼ teaspoon black pepper

½ cup low-fat mayonnaise

3-ounce can Chinese noodles, or ⅓ cup crushed potato chips

Preheat oven to 400°. Slice eggs and arrange on bottom of a large casserole. Mix all the other ingredients except noodles, and pour over the eggs. Top with the noodles or potato chips. Bake at 400° for 30 minutes.

YIELD: 8 SERVINGS
SERVING SIZE: ¾ CUP
CALORIES: 225
EXCHANGES: 1 STARCH/BREAD; 1 MEAT; 1 VEGETABLE; 1 FAT

Eggless Salad

1 cup liquid egg substitute
5 tablespoons low-fat mayonnaise
2 teaspoons minced green onion
½ teaspoon prepared mustard
2 teaspoons minced celery
1 tablespoon minced onion
dash of red pepper
dash of black pepper

Cook egg substitute in a nonstick skillet, covered, over very low heat for 10 minutes, or until the mixture is thickened and set. Remove from heat and cool slightly. Dice the egg substitute. Combine with the remaining ingredients. Chill and serve.

YIELD: 4 SERVINGS
SERVING SIZE: ¼ CUP
CALORIES: 40
EXCHANGE: 1 FAT

Chicken Salad à la King

❦

16-ounce can peach halves in their own juice, drained; reserve juice

1 cup diced cooked chicken

1 rib celery, chopped fine

½ cup frozen peas, thawed

1 tablespoon pimiento

1 small (4 servings) package sugar-free lemon gelatin

1 teaspoon instant chicken bouillon granules

1 cup ice water

nonstick vegetable spray

Garnish

salad greens

½ cup low-fat mayonnaise

½ teaspoon curry powder

2 hard-boiled eggs, sliced

1. Slice peaches, reserving 6 slices for garnish. Chill peaches, chicken, and vegetables.
2. Add enough water to reserved juice to make 1 cup. Bring juice to boiling; remove from hear. Gradually add gelatin to hot juice, stirring constantly until dissolved.
3. Dissolve chicken bouillon in hot liquid, add ice water, peas, celery, pimiento, and peach slices except those reserved for garnish. Pour into a 9-inch pie plate sprayed with nonstick vegetable spray. Chill until firm.

4. To serve, cut into 6 wedges. Line 6 plates with greens and place a wedge of salad on top. Add a dollop of mayonnaise mixed with curry powder. Garnish with reserved peach slices and hard-boiled egg.

YIELD: 6 SERVINGS
SERVING SIZE: 1 WEDGE
CALORIES: 252
EXCHANGES: ½ STARCH/
BREAD; 1 FRUIT; 2 LEAN
MEAT; 1 FAT

12 G FAT
3 G FIBER
14 G PROTEIN
22 G CARBOHYDRATES

469 MG SODIUM
384 MG POTASSIUM
87 MG CHOLESTEROL

Chicken Salad Amandine

4-ounce package slivered almonds
1 cup cubed cooked chicken
10-ounce package frozen peas, thawed
¾ cup sliced celery
1 tablespoon minced onion
2 teaspoons lemon juice
¾ cup nonfat ranch salad dressing

Spread almonds on a nonstick baking sheet and toast in a 350° oven for 8 to 10 minutes. Cool. Combine chicken, peas, almonds, celery, onion, and lemon juice in a bowl. Add dressing and toss.

YIELD: 5 SERVINGS
SERVING SIZE: ¾ CUP
CALORIES: 165
EXCHANGES: 3 LEAN MEAT; 1 VEGETABLE; 2 FAT

A Taste of Slaw

❧

½ head cabbage, shredded

½ cup red bell pepper, cut into thin strips

1 medium carrot, sliced

1 rib celery, chopped

2 green onions, sliced

½ clove garlic, minced

⅛ teaspoon celery seed

2 ounces Provolone cheese, thinly sliced

Dressing

1 cup nonfat plain yogurt

1 teaspoon lemon juice

1 teaspoon Dijon mustard

½ teaspoon salt

⅛ teaspoon pepper

Combine all salad ingredients in a bowl. Combine all ingredients for dressing; pour over vegetables and toss. Chill for 3 hours.

YIELD: 8 SERVINGS	2 G FAT	171 MG SODIUM
SERVING SIZE: ½ CUP	1 G FIBER	214 MG POTASSIUM
CALORIES: 58	4 G PROTEIN	7 MG CHOLESTEROL
EXCHANGES: 1	6 G CARBOHYDRATES	
VEGETABLE; ½ FAT		

German Potato Salad

Our German and Scandinavian friends have served this at many potlucks, parties, and picnics, and I serve it often at home. It is different, refreshing, and can be served either hot or cold. When I became a diabetic I replaced most of the sugar with sugar substitute.

½ pound lean bacon
1 onion, chopped
½ cup flour
½ cup vinegar
½ cup water
2 tablespoons sugar
4 packets sugar substitute
½ teaspoon salt
5 cooked potatoes, sliced

Cube bacon and fry until crisp. Drain. Sauté onion in some of the bacon drippings. Sprinkle with flour over bacon and onions. Stir in vinegar, water, sugar, and sugar substitute. (These ingredients can be adjusted to taste.) Add salt. Bring to a boil. Pour dressing over potatoes and mix well. Can be served hot or warm.

YIELD: 6 SERVINGS
SERVING SIZE: ½ CUP
CALORIES: 150
EXCHANGES: 2 VEGETABLE; 1½ FAT

Savory Salad Dressing

½ cup tomato juice

½ teaspoon steak sauce

2 teaspoons chopped onion

3 tablespoons lemon juice

¼ teaspoon caraway seeds

Combine all ingredients in a jar. Cover and shake well. Chill. Store in refrigerator.

YIELD: 12 TABLESPOONS   0 G FAT   0 G CHOLESTEROL
SERVING SIZE: 1 TABLESPOON
CALORIES: 5.5
EXCHANGES: LESS THAN 20 CALORIES IS A FREE FOOD

Deviled Dressing

6-ounce can vegetable juice cocktail

1 tablespoon safflower or corn oil

1 teaspoon vinegar

½ teaspoon dry mustard

dash of red pepper

Combine all ingredients in a jar. Cover and shake well. Store in refrigerator.

YIELD: ¾ CUP   0 G CHOLESTEROL
SERVING SIZE: 1 TABLESPOON
CALORIES: 13.3 PER SERVING
EXCHANGES: LESS THAN 20 CALORIES IS A FREE FOOD

Orange Dressing

½ cup fresh orange juice

¼ cup fresh lemon juice

½ teaspoon paprika

⅛ teaspoon pepper

½ teaspoon garlic powder

Combine all ingredients in a jar. Cover and shake well. Store in refrigerator.

YIELD: ¾ CUP   0 G FAT   0 G SODIUM

SERVING SIZE: 1 TABLESPOON   0 G CHOLESTEROL

CALORIES: 58

Garlic Croutons

2 slices bread
2 teaspoons margarine, melted
paprika, as desired
garlic powder, as desired

Preheat oven to 300°. Cut bread into ½-inch cubes. Pour melted margarine into shallow baking pan. Add bread cubes and stir lightly to coat. Sprinkle with paprika and garlic powder. Bake at 300° 20 minutes or until cubes are browned and dry. Store in an airtight container for use on soups and salads.

YIELD: 1½ CUPS
SERVING SIZE: 2 TABLESPOONS
CALORIES: 18
EXCHANGES: UP TO 2
TABLESPOONS IS A FREE FOOD

0.8 G FAT
0.1 G FIBER
0.4 G PROTEIN
2.3 G CARBOHYDRATES

31 MG SODIUM
5.2 MG POTASSIUM

MEATS

Meatloaf

❦

1½ pounds lean ground beef, ground turkey, or ground chicken

1 cup bread crumbs

2 eggs, or ½ cup egg substitute

⅓ cup chopped onion

1 teaspoon oregano

1 teaspoon garlic powder

½ teaspoon celery powder

6 tablespoons catsup

Preheat oven to 375°. In a large bowl, combine ground meat, bread crumbs, eggs, onion, oregano, garlic powder, celery powder, and catsup. Shape into a loaf to fit a 9-by-5-inch loaf pan. Cover. Bake at 375° for 45 minutes. Remove cover and bake 10 to 15 minutes longer.

YIELD: 8 SERVINGS
SERVING SIZE: 1 3-OUNCE SLICE

PER SERVING:	BEEF	TURKEY	CHICKEN
CALORIES	215	190	205
TOTAL FAT	9 G	7 G	8 G
SATURATED FAT	4 G	2 G	2 G
FIBER	1 G	1 G	1 G
SODIUM	225 MG	235 MG	230 MG
CHOLESTEROL	53 MG	63 MG	71 MG

Barbecue Beef Bake

❦

1 pound lean ground beef
¾ cup chopped onion
18-ounce bottle barbecue sauce
2 cups shredded low-fat cheddar cheese
2 cups low-fat baking mix, such as Bisquick™
2 eggs
1 cup low-fat (2 percent) milk

Heat oven to 350°. In a skillet, sauté ground beef with ½ cup of the onion until beef is brown. Drain off fat. Stir in barbecue sauce. Pour into an ungreased 9-by-13-inch pan. Sprinkle with cheese. In a bowl, stir baking mix, eggs, and milk until well blended. Spoon over meat mixture. Sprinkle with remaining onion. Bake at 350° for 35 minutes.

YIELD: 9 SERVINGS
SERVING SIZE: 3 OUNCES
CALORIES: 230
EXCHANGES: 1 STARCH/BREAD; 1½ MEAT; 1 FAT

Chopped Ground Beef Steak

※

1 pound lean ground beef
10¾-ounce can cream of mushroom soup, condensed
⅓ cup dry seasoned bread crumbs
1 egg, beaten
¼ cup chopped onion
1 tablespoon cooking oil
1 cup sliced mushrooms (optional)

In a bowl, mix together the ground beef, ½ of the can of soup, bread crumbs, egg, and onions. Shape into 6 patties. In a large frying pan, sauté patties in cooking oil until brown. Drain. Stir together the remaining soup and mushrooms. Pour over the patties, cover and simmer for 25 to 30 minutes, turning once or twice.

YIELD: 6 SERVINGS
SERVING SIZE: 4 OUNCES
CALORIES: 225
EXCHANGE: 2 LEAN MEAT;
½ VEGETABLE, IF MUSHROOMS ARE USED; 1 FAT

Burritos

❦

1 pound lean ground beef
½ cup chopped onion
½ cup chopped green pepper
10-ounce can tomato sauce
8-ounce can whole kernel corn
8 flour tortillas
6 ounces low-fat mozzarella cheese, grated or shredded

1. Sauté meat, onion, and green pepper in a skillet until meat is browned. Drain off fat and return mixture to stove. Add tomato sauce and corn and let simmer 5 to 6 minutes.

2. Preheat oven to 350° While the beef mixture is cooking, soften tortillas according to package directions. Place tortillas in a single layer on a baking sheet. Add spoonfuls of beef mixture to each tortilla and top with cheese. Fold burritos over and secure with a toothpick. Bake at 350° for 8 to 10 minutes.

YIELD: 8 SERVINGS
SERVING SIZE: 1 BURRITO
CALORIES: 200
EXCHANGES: 1 STARCH/BREAD; 1 MEAT; 1 VEGETABLE; 1 FAT

Machaca (Shredded Meat)

2 medium onions, chopped
½ can diced mild green peppers
1 teaspoon crushed red chili flakes
¼ teaspoon cumin
½ teaspoon pepper
½ teaspoon Tabasco™ sauce
1 cup diced canned tomatoes
1 pound beef round steak, cut into pieces

1. Sauté onions, peppers, spices, and sauce in a skillet for 15 minutes. Add tomatoes with their liquid and stir well. Cook for 5 minutes. (Not much liquid will remain.) Add beef. Reduce heat to simmer, cover pan, and cook for 1½ hours or until beef is tender. Refrigerate overnight.
2. Next day: Shred beef pieces using fingers. Reheat over low heat and serve. Very good rolled in tortillas.

YIELD: 6 SERVINGS   4 G FAT   80 MG CHOLESTEROL
SERVING SIZE: 4 OUNCES
CALORIES: 219

Beef Cheese Cups

❧

1 pound ground beef

2 tablespoons chopped onion

2 drops Tabasco™ sauce

1 egg

⅓ cup skim milk

½ cup crushed cheese-flavored crackers

¼ teaspoon salt

1 tablespoon chopped green pepper

dash of black pepper

2 tablespoons chili sauce

nonstick vegetable spray

Preheat oven to 350°. Thoroughly mix all ingredients in a bowl. Coat muffin pan with vegetable spray. Divide meat into 8 balls and place in muffin wells. Bake 40 to 45 minutes.

YIELD: 8 SERVINGS
SERVING SIZE: 1 BEEF CUP
CALORIES: 195

13.7 G FAT
0.3 G FIBER
11.9 G PROTEIN
5 G CARBOHYDRATES

227 MG SODIUM
198 MG POTASSIUM
80 MG CHOLESTEROL

Ground Beef Stroganoff

🌿

1½ pounds lean ground beef
¼ cup chopped onion
¼ cup chopped celery
2 tablespoons chopped green pepper
10¾-ounce can cream of mushroom soup, condensed
¼ soup can of water
8 ounces "lite" sour cream

In a skillet, sauté ground beef, onion, celery, and green pepper until beef is browned. Simmer for 3 minutes, until vegetables are tender. Add the cream of mushroom soup with water, and stir. Add the sour cream and bring to a boil. Serve with rice, noodles, or potatoes.

YIELD: 6 SERVINGS
SERVING SIZE: 4 OUNCES
CALORIES: 150
EXCHANGES: 2½ MEAT; FREE VEGETABLES; 1½ FAT

Meatballs (Scandinavian Style)

I make these several times a year and freeze them. They freeze well and can be used in many different recipes: with gravy, cream of mushroom soup, or tomato sauce, in a casserole, or as a main dish. (*Note:* I have the onions ground with the meat at the store.)

8 pounds ground beef
2 pounds ground pork
6 onions, grind with meat
2 handfuls uncooked oatmeal, or ⅔ cup
3½ cups bread crumbs
6 eggs
3 teaspoons pepper
6 teaspoons salt
3 scant teaspoons nutmeg

Preheat oven to 350°. Mix all ingredients together, very well. Form into walnut-size meatballs. Place on baking sheets, and bake at 350° for 12 to 15 minutes or until brown.

YIELD: APPROX. 150 MEATBALLS
SERVING SIZE: 3 MEATBALLS
CALORIES: 160
EXCHANGES: 1 STARCH/BREAD; 2 MEAT

English Muffin Pizza Melt

1½ pounds lean ground beef

¼ cup chopped onions

nonstick vegetable spray

8-ounce can pizza sauce

¼ teaspoon garlic powder

½ teaspoon basil

1 teaspoon parsley flakes

3 plain English muffins, split

2 tablespoons shredded mozzarella cheese

Preheat oven to 350°. In a skillet sprayed with nonstick vegetable spray, cook beef and onion until meat is browned. Drain off fat and pat with paper towels. Stir in pizza sauce and seasonings. Top each muffin half with 3 tablespoons beef mixture and 1 teaspoon cheese. (Muffins may be pretoasted before adding meat and cheese.) Bake at 350° for 12 to 15 minutes or until heated through and cheese is melted.

YIELD: 6 SERVINGS	12 G FAT	497 MG SODIUM
SERVING SIZE: ½ MUFFIN	1 G FIBER	488 MG POTASSIUM
AND 3 TABLESPOONS	17 G PROTEIN	50 MG CHOLESTEROL
BEEF TOPPING	17 G CARBOHYDRATES	
CALORIES: 244		

Sloppy Joe Pitas

nonstick vegetable spray
1¼ pounds lean ground beef
¼ cup chopped onion
¼ cup chopped green pepper
8-ounce can tomato sauce
½ teaspoon onion powder
¼ teaspoon black pepper
½ teaspoon garlic powder
½ teaspoon salt
2 large pitas

Spray large skillet with nonstick vegetable spray. Cook ground beef, onion, and green pepper until meat is browned. Drain off fat and pat dry with paper towels. Stir in tomato sauce and seasonings. Cook until heated thoroughly (about 10 minutes), stirring several times. Cut pitas in half and stuff each half with ½ cup meat mixture. (Pitas may be crisped in warm oven before stuffing.)

YIELD: 4 SERVINGS	15 G FAT	839 MG SODIUM
SERVING SIZE: ½ PITA	2 G FIBER	515 MG POTASSIUM
PLUS ½ CUP FILLING	24 G PROTEIN	75 MG CHOLESTEROL
CALORIES: 302	17 G CARBOHYDRATES	

Pot Roast with Vegetables

1½ pounds lean boneless chuck roast

nonstick vegetable spray

1 large onion, peeled and sliced

¼ cup chopped celery

½ cup water

¼ teaspoon salt

¼ teaspoon pepper

4 large carrots, peeled and sliced

2 or 3 potatoes, peeled and sliced

1. Brown chuck roast over medium heat in a dutch oven coated with vegetable spray. Add onion, celery, water, salt, and pepper.
2. Cover dutch oven and bake at 350° for 1 hour and 20 minutes. Add sliced carrots and potatoes and continue to bake covered for 1 hour or until meat and vegetables are tender.
3. Place meat and vegetables on a serving platter and slice meat.

YIELD: 8 SERVINGS
SERVING SIZE: ½ CUP
CALORIES: 200
EXCHANGES: 2 MEAT; 2 VEGETABLE

Swiss Steak

❦

2 tablespoons flour
½ teaspoon salt
¼ teaspoon pepper
⅛ teaspoon meat tenderizer
1 pound round steak, cut into serving pieces
2 tablespoons margarine
10¾-ounce can cream of mushroom soup, condensed
½ soup can water

1. Mix flour, salt, pepper, and meat tenderizer, and pound into each piece of meat. Melt the margarine in a frying pan and brown the steak.
2. Preheat oven to 300°. Place meat in a baking dish. Pour the mushroom soup and water over the meat and bake at 300° for about 2½ hours or until tender.

YIELD: 4 SERVINGS
SERVING SIZE: 4 OUNCES
CALORIES: 230
EXCHANGES: 2 MEAT; 1 FAT

Frikadeller (Danish Meatballs)

The recipe for frikadeller comes from both my mother's and father's sides of the family. My paternal grandmother always made them with beef and pork. My maternal grandmother sometimes made them with beef alone. They puff up so they're soft on the inside, crispy on the outside, and delicious. I remember my mother mixing frikadeller with her hands, and I find that I often do that, too.

1 pound lean ground beef
½ pound lean ground pork
¼ cup flour
1 onion, grated
1 teaspoon salt
½ teaspoon pepper
2 eggs
¾ cup low-fat (2 percent) milk
1 teaspoon margarine

Mix meat in a bowl with flour, onion, salt, and pepper. Add eggs, one at a time, then the milk. Mix well. Form into 8 or 10 patties. Fry in margarine in a heavy skillet over medium heat for 45 minutes, turning often.

YIELD: 8 TO 10 PATTIES
SERVING SIZE: 1 PATTY
CALORIES: 220
EXCHANGES: 2 MEAT; 1 FAT

Beef Sausage

2 pounds lean ground beef

1 tablespoon meat tenderizer

½ cup water

½ teaspoon liquid smoke

¼ teaspoon garlic powder

¼ teaspoon pepper

1 tablespoon mustard seed

Mix all ingredients. Roll into 4 sausage-shaped logs. Wrap individually in foil and chill overnight. To cook, poke holes in foil to allow liquid to drain. Place foil-covered sausages on a rack over a baking pan. Bake at 350° for 1 hour. Cut each sausage into 10 slices.

YIELD: 40 SLICES   6 G FAT   35 MG CHOLESTEROL
SERVING SIZE: 3 SLICES   15 G PROTEIN
CALORIES: 114   0 G CARBOHYDRATES

Taco Casserole

❦

We like taco salads; one day I thought, why not a taco casserole made to taste like a taco salad without the lettuce? I began to experiment, and the first efforts failed for one reason or another. But I persisted and finally got it right. Some people prefer less taco seasoning; adjust the seasoning accordingly.

8-ounce package medium-width noodles, such as fettuccine
1½ to 2 pounds lean ground beef
¼ cup diced onion
2 tablespoons diced celery
2 tablespoons diced green pepper
¼ cup "lite" sour cream
1 package taco seasoning mix
28-ounce can stewed tomatoes

1. Boil noodles per package directions. Drain and set aside.
2. In a skillet, brown ground beef and drain off fat. Add onion, celery, green pepper, and sour cream. Simmer for 10 to 12 minutes.
3. Preheat oven to 350°. Transfer meat mixture to a large casserole dish. Add noodles to the meat mixture. Add package of taco seasoning and stewed tomatoes. Stir until well blended. Bake at 350° for 45 minutes to 1 hour, until hot and bubbly.

YIELD: 5 CUPS; 10 SERVINGS
SERVING SIZE: ½ CUP
CALORIES: 240
EXCHANGES: 1 STARCH/BREAD; 2 MEAT; 1 VEGETABLE; 1 FAT

Dijon Chicken

2 tablespoons "lite" margarine

½ clove garlic, crushed

2 whole boneless, skinless chicken breasts

½ cup white grape juice

½ cup water

2 tablespoons Dijon mustard

½ teaspoon dillweed

½ teaspoon salt

¼ teaspoon black pepper

⅓ cup crushed fresh parsley

1. Preheat oven to 325°. Heat margarine in a large frying pan, add garlic, and cook 2 minutes over medium heat. In same pan, brown chicken pieces 3 minutes on each side. Transfer chicken to a large casserole.

2. Add the grape juice, water, mustard, dillweed, salt, and pepper to the frying pan and stir to mix with the chicken drippings. Bring to a boil and cook for 2 minutes. Pour over chicken in the casserole. Cover and bake at 325° for 30 minutes. Add parsley, baste the chicken with the sauce, and bake for 5 minutes longer.

YIELD: 4 SERVINGS	2 G FAT	235 MG SODIUM
SERVING SIZE: ½ BREAST	1 G FIBER	72 MG CHOLESTEROL
PLUS 2 TABLESPOONS SAUCE	27 G PROTEIN	
CALORIES: 225	2 G CARBOHYDRATES	

Chicken Marengo

🌱

nonstick vegetable spray
2½ pounds boneless, skinless chicken
4 ounces pound fresh mushrooms, sliced
2 onions, sliced
28-ounce can tomatoes, slightly crushed with juice
½ cup white grape juice
½ teaspoon garlic powder
½ teaspoon salt
⅛ teaspoon black pepper

Preheat oven to 350°. Spray a large ovenproof pan with nonstick cooking spray. Sauté chicken until brown on all sides, about 15 minutes. Add mushrooms, onions, tomatoes with juice, grape juice, and seasonings. Stir into chicken. Cover with foil and bake at 350° for 1 to 1½ hours or until tender.

YIELD: 4 SERVINGS   9 G FAT   689 MG SODIUM
SERVING SIZE: 5 OUNCES   5 G FIBER   1,003 MG POTASSIUM
CHICKEN PLUS ½ CUP   16 G CARBOHYDRATES   95 MG CHOLESTEROL
SAUCE
CALORIES: 279

Easy Mexican Fajitas

6 flour tortillas

2 tablespoons cooking oil

1 medium green pepper, cut into rings or strips

1 medium red pepper, cut into rings or strips

1 medium onion, cut into rings

*1 oven-roasted chicken or turkey breast, cut into strips ¼ inch
wide(about 1 to 1¼ pounds of meat)*

1 teaspoon Cajun seasoning, or 1 tablespoon chili powder

1½ cups shredded lettuce

1½ cups chopped fresh tomatoes

Heat tortillas in oven or microwave. In a 12-inch skillet, over
medium heat, sauté green and red peppers and onion in oil for 2
minutes. Add chicken or turkey strips and Cajun seasoning, stirring to coat. Cover and heat through for 5 minutes. Fill each tortilla with the chicken mixture, then add lettuce and tomatoes.

YIELD: 6 SERVINGS 8 G FAT (20% CALORIES FROM FAT)
SERVING SIZE: 1 TORTILLA 837 MG SODIUM
AND APPROX. 3 OUNCES MEAT 15 MG CHOLESTEROL
CALORIES: 253

Chicken Bits

¼ *cup margarine*

½ *cup chicken bouillon*

2 tablespoons chopped celery

1 teaspoon chopped fresh parsley

½ *cup flour*

2 eggs

½ *cup finely chopped cooked chicken*

2 tablespoons toasted almonds, slivered

1. Preheat oven to 400°. In a skillet, cook margarine and bouillon over medium heat until margarine is melted. Stir in celery, parsley, and flour. Continue cooking until mixture forms a ball in the middle of the pan. Cool for 10 minutes.

2. Add eggs, one at a time, beating until mixture is shiny. Add chicken and almonds. Drop by teaspoons on ungreased baking sheet. Bake at 400° for 15 to 20 minutes.

YIELD: 30 BITS	4 G FAT	82 MG SODIUM
SERVING SIZE: 2 BITS	4 G PROTEIN	42 MG CHOLESTEROL
CALORIES: 70	4 G CARBOHYDRATES	

Lemon Chicken

❦

We serve this often in our home and take it to picnics and potlucks. It is one of the recipes my friends have elected "a keeper."

⅓ cup lemon juice
½ clove garlic, minced
¼ cup reduced-sodium soy sauce
½ teaspoon ginger
½ teaspoon salt
½ teaspoon pepper
2 pounds boneless, skinless chicken breasts
nonstick vegetable spray

1. In a mixing bowl, combine lemon juice, garlic, soy sauce, ginger, salt, and pepper, stirring until well mixed. Add chicken, cover, and marinate for 3 to 4 hours in the refrigerator, turning once.
2. Drain and discard marinade. Transfer chicken to a shallow roasting pan, coated with vegetable spray. Bake at 325° for 1 hour or until chicken is done.

YIELD: 10 SERVINGS
SERVING SIZE: 1 SLICE, 3½ OUNCES
CALORIES: 75

1 G FAT
15 G PROTEIN
1 G CARBOHYDRATES

306 MG SODIUM
37 MG CHOLESTEROL

Baked Chicken

This recipe is also popular at potlucks, picnics, and dinners. I often bake the chicken breasts and place them in the freezer (they freeze well) to be used later as a base for a casserole, salad, or as an entrée. This dish was also voted "a keeper" by our friends.

4 chicken skinless, boneless breasts
1 teaspoon onion powder
1 teaspoon garlic powder
1 teaspoon celery powder
¼ teaspoon paprika
¼ teaspoon black pepper
½ teaspoon oregano
½ teaspoon basil
2 tablespoons lemon juice
2 tablespoons water

Preheat oven to 350°. Place chicken breasts in a 9-by-13-inch baking pan. Mix spices together and sprinkle over chicken. Mix lemon juice and water and pour over chicken. Bake at 350° for 1 hour. May be served at once or frozen for later use.

YIELD: 8 SERVINGS
SERVING SIZE: ½ BREAST
CALORIES: 300

Chicken à la King

2 chicken bouillon cubes

1½ cups hot water

3 tablespoons margarine

3 tablespoons flour

2½ cups diced cooked chicken

1 cup cooked peas

½ cup sliced cooked carrots

¼ cup chopped onion

4-ounce can sliced mushrooms, drained

2 tablespoons chopped pimientos

1 teaspoon salt

Dissolve bouillon cubes in hot water. Stir well. In a saucepan, melt margarine and blend in flour. Add broth slowly, stirring constantly. Cook over medium heat until mixture thickens, stirring constantly to prevent lumps. Add other ingredients, stir, and heat until mixture comes to a boil and begins to bubble. Serve over rice or biscuits—remember to add the necessary bread exchanges and calories.

YIELD: 6 CUPS;	7.8 G FAT	780 MG SODIUM
8 SERVINGS	2.1 G FIBER	211 MG POTASSIUM
SERVING SIZE: ¾ CUP	14.8 G PROTEIN	39 MG CHOLESTEROL
CALORIES: 165	8.2 G CARBOHYDRATES	

Chicken Nuggets with Barbecue Dipping Sauce

2 whole boneless, skinless chicken breasts
(about 1 pound), cut into 12 cubes
½ teaspoon salt
¼ teaspoon pepper
1 egg, beaten
½ cup dry bread crumbs

Barbecue Sauce
2 tablespoons catsup
2 tablespoons prepared mustard
½ teaspoon minced onion flakes
1 teaspoon brown sugar substitute
1 teaspoon Worcestershire sauce

Preheat oven to 350°. Sprinkle chicken nuggets with salt and pepper. Dip nuggets in beaten egg, then in bread crumbs. Place on a cookie sheet. Bake at 350° for 20 to 25 minutes or until lightly browned and juices run clear.

For sauce: Combine catsup, mustard, onion, brown sugar substitute, and Worcestershire sauce, and mix well. Serve with nuggets, about 1 tablespoon of sauce per serving. Or, instead of barbecue sauce, try low-salt teriyaki, sweet-and-sour sauce, or hot mustard sauce.

YIELD: 12 NUGGETS,   5 G FAT   358 MG SODIUM
⅓ CUP SAUCE   0 G FIBER   302 MG POTASSIUM
SERVING SIZE: 3   30 G PROTEIN   140 MG CHOLESTEROL
NUGGETS PLUS APPROX.   12 G CARBOHYDRATES
1 TABLESPOON OF SAUCE
CALORIES: 225

Spicy Turkey Roast

❦

1 whole boneless, rolled turkey breast (4 pounds), thawed

6 large cloves garlic

3 tablespoons rosemary

1 tablespoon black pepper

¼ teaspoon red pepper

1 teaspoon paprika

1 teaspoon salt

2 tablespoons cooking oil

1. Remove mesh from the turkey. Lay out as flat as possible on cutting board, placing the skin side down. Combine the garlic, rosemary, black pepper, red pepper, paprika, and salt in a bowl (a food processor or a blender works very well). Add the oil and mix very well, until coarsely chopped. Spread half of this mixture over the inside of the turkey.

2. Preheat oven to 375°. Re-roll the turkey to its original log shape, tying firmly with string. Spread evenly with the remaining spice mixture. Place on a rack in a roasting pan, and roast at 375° for 1½ to 2 hours, until a meat thermometer registers 170°. (A long log shape takes less time then a compact roast.) Remove from oven.

3. Let roast stand for 10 minutes before slicing thinly. Garnish with rosemary if desired. Scrape up cooking juices from bot-

tom of pan and spoon over meat, or thicken with flour and add chicken broth for a gravy.

YIELD: 10 SLICES
SERVING SIZE: 5 OUNCES
CALORIES: 264

9.7 G FAT
40 G PROTEIN
2 G CARBOHYDRATES

331 MG SODIUM

Tomatoey Baked Chicken

nonstick vegetable spray
4 boneless, skinless chicken breast halves, about 3 ounces each
12-ounce can whole tomatoes, drained and chopped
½ cup chopped onion
½ cup chopped green pepper
½ teaspoon garlic powder
¼ teaspoon dried oregano
¼ teaspoon dried basil
¼ teaspoon pepper

Preheat oven to 400°. Coat a baking dish with cooking spray and arrange chicken in it. Combine tomatoes and remaining ingredients, stirring until well combined. Spoon over chicken. Cover and bake at 400° for 1 hour.

YIELD: 4 SERVINGS
SERVING SIZE: ½ BREAST
WITH ¼ CUP OF SAUCE
CALORIES: 96

1 G FAT
1 G FIBER
15 G PROTEIN
6 G CARBOHYDRATES

207 MG SODIUM
48 MG CHOLESTEROL

Chicken with Vegetables and Rice

1 boneless, skinless chicken breast, thinly sliced

1 small onion, chopped

4-ounce can mushrooms, drained (optional)

1 teaspoon canola oil

18-ounce can chop suey vegetables, drained and rinsed

6 ounces chicken broth

½ cup water

2 teaspoons soy sauce

1½ tablespoons cornstarch

½ teaspoon ginger

1 cup uncooked rice

1. In a skillet, sauté the chicken breast, onion, and mushrooms in the canola oil for 2 minutes. Add chop suey vegetables.
2. In a saucepan, combine chicken broth, water, soy sauce, cornstarch, and ginger over medium heat, stirring constantly until thickened. Add to the chicken and vegetable mixture. Cook until the cornstarch is thickened, smooth, and not lumpy.
3. Boil rice as directed on package. Serve chicken mixture over the hot rice; or combine chicken and rice in a casserole and bake at 350° for 30 minutes.

YIELD: 4 SERVINGS   3 G FAT
SERVING SIZE: 1 CUP
CALORIES: 250
EXCHANGES: 1 MEAT; 1½ VEGETABLE; 1 FAT

Chicken Glazed with Citrus Fruit

8-ounce can pineapple slices, in their own juice
2 tablespoons "lite" margarine
1 tablespoon lemon juice
1 teaspoon grated lemon peel
1 teaspoon grated orange peel
5 cut-up boneless chicken breasts, 1½ to 1¾ pounds
orange slices for garnish

1. Drain the pineapple, reserving ¼ cup juice. Set pineapple and juice aside. For citrus glaze, melt margarine and stir in reserved ¼ cup pineapple juice, lemon juice, and lemon and orange peels. Set aside.

2. Place the chicken pieces, skin side down, on the rack on an unheated broiler pan. Place under broiler and broil 5 to 6 inches from heat about 20 minutes until lightly browned. Brush chicken pieces with citrus glaze. Turn pieces skin side up and broil for 15 to 20 minutes more, or until tender, brushing with glaze occasionally. Add pineapple slices to broiler rack the last 5 minutes.

3. Remove the chicken pieces and pineapple slices from the broiler rack. Garnish with orange slices.

Yield: 6 servings
Serving size: 4 to 5 ounces chicken
Calories: 285
Exchanges: 1½ Fruit; 2 Meat; 1 Fat

Sauerkraut and Pork Chops

1 pound lean center-cut pork chops
2 cups sauerkraut, drained
1 small apple, peeled and sliced
1 teaspoon caraway seeds (optional)

Preheat oven to 350°. Brown pork chops in a skillet. Mix sauerkraut with meat juices in skillet. Layer half of sauerkraut, half of apple slices, and half of caraway seeds in large casserole. Place pork chops over mixture. Layer remaining sauerkraut, apples, and caraway seeds. Cover and bake at 350° for 1 hour and 45 minutes, or until pork is tender. (*Note:* This dish is not for low-sodium diets.)

YIELD: 4 SERVINGS
SERVING SIZE: 1 CHOP
AND ½ CUP SAUERKRAUT
MIXTURE
CALORIES: 215

10.7 G FAT
2.9 G FIBER
21.2 G PROTEIN
9 G CARBOHYDRATES

832.2 MG SODIUM
504.5 MG POTASSIUM
67 MG CHOLESTEROL

Barbecued Spareribs

🌿

2 pounds pork spareribs

1 tablespoon margarine

½ medium onion, minced

1 small clove garlic, minced

1 cup catsup, or chili sauce, or some of each

2 tablespoons brown sugar substitute

1 teaspoon Worcestershire sauce

1 teaspoon prepared mustard

6 drops Tabasco™ sauce

¼ teaspoon pepper

1 teaspoon lemon juice

1. Cook ribs over charcoals (or in oven at 300°) until well done, about 2 hours, basting frequently with water to keep spareribs moist.

2. Melt margarine in a medium saucepan. Sauté onion and garlic in margarine until tender, about 5 minutes. Add remaining ingredients except lemon juice. Simmer for 10 minutes, then add lemon juice.

3. Brush sauce onto ribs during last 5 minutes of cooking, or serve with ribs for dipping.

YIELD: 8 SERVINGS
SERVING SIZE: ¼ POUND
RIBS PLUS 2 TABLESPOONS
SAUCE
CALORIES: 238
EXCHANGES: ½ STARCH/
BREAD; 2 MEDIUM-FAT
MEAT; 1 FAT

15 G FAT
0 G FIBER
14 G PROTEIN
12 G CARBOHYDRATES

430 MG SODIUM
284 MG POTASSIUM
53 MG CHOLESTEROL

Barbecued Pork

8-ounce can tomato sauce

1 teaspoon Worcestershire sauce

1 teaspoon prepared yellow mustard

1 teaspoon minced dried onion flakes

½ teaspoon brown sugar substitute

¼ teaspoon garlic powder

4 dashes Tabasco™ sauce (or to taste)

1 pound cooked boneless pork, thinly sliced

Combine all ingredients except pork in a 10-inch skillet. Bring to a boil and reduce heat to simmer. Add pork slices and stir well to coat. Cover and heat for 5 minutes or until heated thoroughly. Serve as an entrée or on buns for sandwiches.

YIELD: 4 SERVINGS   16 G FAT   450 MG SODIUM
SERVING SIZE: 4 OUNCES   1 G FIBER   642 MG POTASSIUM
PORK PLUS SAUCE,   4 G CARBOHYDRATES   102 MG CHOLESTEROL
WITHOUT BUN
CALORIES: 293
EXCHANGES: 4 LEAN MEAT;
1 VEGETABLE; 1 FAT

Diet Salmon Loaf

15-ounce can salmon, drained, bones and skin removed

2 eggs, separated

½ cup low-fat (2 percent) milk

¼ cup chopped celery

2 tablespoons chopped onion

2 tablespoons parsley flakes

2 teaspoons lemon juice

½ teaspoon salt

dash black pepper

Preheat oven to 350°. In a large bowl, mash salmon with a fork. In separate bowl, beat egg yolks and milk together. Add chopped celery, chopped onion, parsley flakes, lemon juice, salt, and pepper. Add to salmon and mix well. Beat egg whites until stiff. Carefully fold into salmon mixture. Bake in a 9-by-5-inch loaf pan for 45 to 50 minutes at 350°.

YIELD: 5 SERVINGS
SERVING SIZE: 4 OUNCES
CALORIES: 186
EXCHANGES: 3 LEAN MEAT

VEGETABLES

Quick Maple Candied Carrots

🌿

16-ounce can sliced carrots, undrained
1 tablespoon sugar-free maple syrup
2 teaspoons "lite" margarine
dash of lemon juice (optional)
dash of salt and pepper

Heat carrots in saucepan; drain well. Stir in remaining ingredients. Heat through.

YIELD: 2 CUPS
SERVING SIZE: ½ CUP
CALORIES: 53

1.4 G FAT
0.7 G PROTEIN
10.6 G CARBOHYDRATES

286 MG SODIUM
0 MG CHOLESTEROL

Stir-Fried Peppers and Tomatoes

❦

1 green pepper

2 cups cherry tomatoes

2 teaspoons cooking oil

1 tablespoon chopped fresh basil

⅛ teaspoon garlic powder

⅛ teaspoon pepper

Cut green peppers in half lengthwise. Remove seeds, stem, and core. Cut into thin strips and set aside. Remove stems from tomatoes. Cut in half and set aside. In a large skillet, heat oil and cook green pepper strips and basil for 3 minutes. Add cherry tomatoes. Cover and cook for 2 minutes more or until heated through. Sprinkle with garlic powder and pepper.

YIELD: 4 SERVINGS

SERVING SIZE: ¾ CUP

CALORIES: 20

EXCHANGES: ½ VEGETABLE; ½ FAT

Creamed Cucumbers and Onions

2 tablespoons nonfat mayonnaise

¼ cup skim milk

¼ cup vinegar

1 cucumber, thinly sliced

¼ cup chopped onion

½ teaspoon pepper, or to taste

1 teaspoon sugar substitute

Mix together mayonnaise, milk, and vinegar until smooth. Add the cucumber and onion and blend well. Add the pepper (to taste) and the sugar substitute.

YIELD: 3 SERVINGS
SERVING SIZE: ¼ CUP
CALORIES: 20
EXCHANGES: 1 FAT

Pineapple Glazed Yams

*8-ounce can pineapple chunks in their own juice, drained;
reserve juice*

2 teaspoons cornstarch

¼ teaspoon salt

⅛ teaspoon black pepper

⅛ teaspoon cinnamon

*½ pound yams (2 small), cooked, peeled, and sliced ¼-inch thick,
then each slice cut into smaller pieces*

1 teaspoon margarine

Preheat oven to 350°. In a 1½-quart saucepan, combine reserved pineapple juice mixed with cornstarch, salt, pepper, and cinnamon. Cook until thickened, stirring constantly. Combine yams and pineapple in an 8-inch casserole. Stir in sauce and mix well. Dot with margarine. Cover with foil and bake at 350° for 15 to 20 minutes.

YIELD: 4 SERVINGS	1 G FAT	149 MG SODIUM
SERVING SIZE: ¼ CUP	2 G FIBER	399 MG POTASSIUM
CALORIES: 105	1 G PROTEIN	0 MG CHOLESTEROL
	24 G CARBOHYDRATES	

Hash Brown Potato Casserole

*32-ounce package frozen hash brown potatoes,
thawed and broken up*

12-ounce package low-fat cheddar cheese, grated

1 cup "lite" sour cream

10¾-ounce can cream of chicken soup, condensed

½ cup margarine, melted

2 cups Cornflakes™

Preheat oven to 350°. Mix hash brown potatoes, cheddar cheese, sour cream, cream of chicken soup, and margarine (reserve 2 tablespoons) together. Pour into a 9-by-13-inch pan, or into two 9-by-5-inch pans. Mix cornflakes and remainder of melted margarine together and sprinkle on top. Bake at 350° for 45 to 50 minutes. (*Note:* This casserole freezes very well.)

YIELD: 10 SERVINGS	7 G FAT	50 MG SODIUM
SERVING SIZE: 1 CUP	2 G PROTEIN	250 MG POTASSIUM
CALORIES: 250	25 G CARBOHYDRATES	30 MG CHOLESTEROL

Sliced Baked Potatoes

4 medium potatoes

1 teaspoon salt

3 tablespoons melted margarine

2 to 3 teaspoons chopped fresh herbs, such as parsley, sage, thyme, or chives; or 2 to 3 teaspoons dried herbs of your choice

8 ounces cheddar cheese, grated or shredded

Preheat oven to 425°. Peel potatoes and slice them thinly, but not all the way through. (Use the handle of a spoon or knife to prevent the knife from cutting all the way through.) Place potatoes in a baking dish, fanning slightly. Sprinkle with salt and drizzle margarine over them. Sprinkle with herbs. Cover with foil. Bake potatoes at 425° about 45 minutes. Remove from oven and remove foil. Top each potato with 1 tablespoon grated cheese. Return potatoes to oven and bake for another 15 minutes, or until lightly browned, cheese is melted, and potatoes are soft inside. Check with a fork.

YIELD: 4 SERVINGS   8.5 G FAT   730 MG SODIUM
SERVING SIZE: 1 POTATO   5.6 G PROTEIN
CALORIES: 235   33 G CARBOHYDRATES

Potato "Skins"

1 cup instant mashed potato flakes
1 cup water
1 tablespoon whole-wheat or white flour
1½ cups grated low-fat cheese, such as cheddar or mozzarella
8 slices of lean bacon, crisply cooked, crumbled

1. Prepare instant potatoes as directed on package, except decrease water to 1 cup. Add flour. Refrigerate until cool.
2. Preheat oven to 425°. Form mixture into 16 oval patties. Press on a cookie sheet to ¼ inch thick. Bake at 425° for 25 to 30 minutes. Remove from oven and top with bacon and cheese. Return to oven until cheese melts.

YIELD: 16 PATTIES   4 G FAT   135 MG SODIUM
SERVING SIZE: 1 PATTY   4 G PROTEIN   12 MG CHOLESTEROL
CALORIES: 60   4 G CARBOHYDRATES

Potatoes au Gratin

½ cup low-fat (2 percent) milk
2 tablespoons flour
½ teaspoon salt
⅛ teaspoon celery powder
2 cups unpeeled, thinly sliced potatoes
¾ cup shredded cheddar cheese
2 tablespoons margarine
¼ teaspoon paprika

Preheat oven to 350°. Heat milk in saucepan for 2 minutes, but do not boil. Combine flour, salt, celery powder, and cheese in a small bowl. Place half of the potatoes in an 8-inch square baking pan. Sprinkle half of the cheese over the potatoes. Repeat layers. Pour hot milk over all, then dot with margarine. Sprinkle with paprika. Cover with foil and bake at 350° for 15 to 20 minutes. Uncover and bake for 10 to 15 minutes longer or until potatoes are tender when pricked with a fork.

YIELD: 4 SERVINGS
SERVING SIZE: ½ CUP
CALORIES: 214

9 G FAT
2 G FIBER
9 G PROTEIN
25 G CARBOHYDRATES

440 MG SODIUM
400 MG POTASSIUM
23 MG CHOLESTEROL

German-Style Sauerkraut

1 medium onion, thinly sliced

nonstick vegetable spray

16-ounce can sauerkraut, rinsed and drained

3 slices bacon, cooked crisp and crumbled

1 large apple, peeled, cored, and diced

½ teaspoon caraway seeds

2 cups boiling water

½ teaspoon brown sugar substitute

In a 2-quart saucepan sprayed with nonstick vegetable spray, sauté onion until brown. Add sauerkraut and cook for 5 minutes. Stir in bacon, apple, and caraway seeds. Cover with boiling water. Cook uncovered for 15 minutes over low heat. Stir in brown sugar substitute. Serve with pork chops, sausage, or beef.

YIELD: 4 SERVINGS   3.5 G FIBER   400 MG SODIUM

SERVING SIZE: ½ CUP

CALORIES: 180

Sweet Corn

Select ripe, sweet corn, and season with Molly McButter™. Husk and remove the silk. Wrap in waxed paper. Place in microwave at medium setting for 4 minutes (maximum 8 ears at once). Turn, then microwave for another 4 minutes.

SERVING SIZE: 1 MEDIUM EAR
CALORIES: 132 (WITH 1 TEASPOON MARGARINE)
EXCHANGES: 1 6-INCH EAR = 1 STARCH/BREAD

Sautéed Zucchini

1 medium zucchini
1 tablespoon cooking oil
½ cup chopped onion
dash pepper
dash salt
¼ teaspoon celery powder
¼ teaspoon oregano

Clean zucchini and slice thinly. Heat oil in frying pan and cook onion until browned. Add zucchini and cook for 3 to 4 minutes. Add spices and stir well.

YIELD: 4 SERVINGS
SERVING SIZE: ¼ ZUCCHINI
CALORIES: 58
EXCHANGES: 1 VEGETABLE; ½ FAT

4 G FAT
2 G FIBER
2 G PROTEIN
5 G CARBOHYDRATES

Stuffed Tomatoes

This is another recipe that posed a challenge. The tomatoes kept coming out pasty and tough until I came up with this version. You can substitute green peppers for the tomatoes.

½ pound lean ground beef

2 tablespoons chopped onion

2 tablespoons chopped celery

2 tablespoons chopped green pepper

2 large, firm tomatoes

⅛ teaspoon salt

⅛ teaspoon pepper

2 tablespoons finely grated low-fat cheese,
such as cheddar or mozzarella

Brown ground beef with onion, celery, and green pepper. Halve tomatoes and scoop out centers carefully. Add tomato pulp to the ground beef. Season with salt and pepper and mix well. Fill the tomato shells with the beef mixture and top with the cheese. Place under broiler for 2 to 3 minutes, until hot and bubbly. Watch carefully so they do not burn.

YIELD: 4 SERVINGS
SERVING SIZE: ½ TOMATO WITH STUFFING
CALORIES: 140
EXCHANGES: 2 LEAN MEAT; 1 VEGETABLE

Annette's Cabbage Rolls

My mother had a friend everyone called Nettie. Her name was really Annette; I thought that was such a pretty name. She made the most delicious cabbage rolls and we always enjoyed them at potlucks. I thought it only fitting to name my modified version of this recipe in Annette's honor. I have shared this recipe often and everyone likes them. In fact, I gave the recipe to one of my nutritionists and now they're the only cabbage rolls her family will eat. It's definitely "a keeper"! (*Note:* This dish is not for low-sodium diets.)

1 large head cabbage

1 pound lean ground beef

1 cup uncooked white rice

1 egg

2 tablespoons chopped onion

16-ounce can sauerkraut, drained

8-ounce can tomato sauce

1. Preheat oven to 350°. Remove the core from the cabbage head and pull off 12 leaves. Rinse leaves in cold water. Cut the heavy stem from the base of each leaf and place leaves in a pan of boiling water to soften. Cover pan and turn off heat to steam.

2. Mix ground beef, rice, egg, and chopped onion in a bowl. Remove cabbage from water and place sauerkraut in the same water. Place a heaping teaspoon of beef mixture in the center

of each leaf. Fold over half of leaf, tuck in ends, and roll up. Secure with a toothpick.

3. Remove sauerkraut from the hot water, drain. Layer sauerkraut in a 2-quart casserole. Place each roll, folded side down, on the sauerkraut. Pour tomato sauce over rolls. Cover and bake at 350° for 1 hour.

YIELD: 12 SERVINGS
SERVING SIZE: 1 CABBAGE ROLL
CALORIES: 190
EXCHANGE: 1 MEAT; 2 VEGETABLE; 1 FAT

Ron's Sweet-and-Sour Green Beans

🌿

I had to experiment with this in trying to take the sweetness out of the original recipe. It ended up much too sweet. But I got it right on the third try. Now, it is a favorite dish of my family and friends.

8 strips lean bacon

1 tablespoon brown sugar

¼ teaspoon dried mustard

½ teaspoon salt

⅛ teaspoon black pepper

*brown sugar substitute equal to
1 tablespoon brown sugar*

3 tablespoons vinegar

1 tablespoon water

14.5-ounce can of green beans

paprika to taste

Cook bacon until crisp. Drain off fat and dice. Combine dry ingredients and add to bacon. Add vinegar and water and heat to boiling. Boil 1 minute. Pour over green beans and heat for 2 to 3 minutes. Sprinkle with paprika.

YIELD: 6 SERVINGS
SERVING SIZE: 3½ OUNCES
CALORIES: 140
EXCHANGE: 1 MEAT; 1 VEGETABLE; 2 FAT

Dad C.'s Baked Beans

❧

This was my dad's recipe. He would make a "baking of beans" and share them with family and friends.

2 pounds dried navy beans

1 teaspoon baking soda

1 pound lean bacon

⅔ cup molasses

½ cup catsup

*¼ cup brown sugar, and enough brown sugar
substitute to equal another ¼ cup*

1 medium onion, chopped

2 teaspoons dried mustard

½ teaspoon salt

½ teaspoon black pepper

1. Soak beans overnight in cold water.
2. Next day, drain and add fresh water to cover. Cook beans covered over low heat until tender and a sample bean can be mashed with a fork (about 1½ hours). Add baking soda, let fizz, then drain off liquid.
3. Preheat oven to 300°. Place beans in a large greased roasting pan. Cut bacon into small pieces and add to the beans. Mix in remaining ingredients. Bake at 300° for 6 hours.

YIELD: 40 SERVINGS
SERVING SIZE: ¼ CUP
CALORIES: 94
EXCHANGES: 1 STARCH/BREAD; 1 MEAT; 2 FAT

Broccoli au Gratin

10-ounce package frozen broccoli, cut or chopped
½ of 10.5-ounce can cream of mushroom soup, condensed
¼ cup grated cheddar cheese
1 teaspoon margarine
2 tablespoons dry bread crumbs

Preheat oven to 350°. Cook broccoli until crisp-tender. Drain. Stir in soup and cheese. Turn into a 1-quart baking dish. Melt margarine in small skillet over medium heat. Add bread crumbs and stir until lightly browned. Sprinkle crumbs over casserole. Bake at 350° 30 minutes or until heated through.

YIELD: 2 CUPS   6.3 G FAT   407.7 MG SODIUM
SERVING SIZE: ½ CUP   1.8 G FIBER   156 MG POTASSIUM
CALORIES: 106   44.8 G PROTEIN   8 MG CHOLESTEROL
EXCHANGES: 2 VEGETABLE;   8.6 G CARBOHYDRATES
1 FAT

CASSEROLES AND OTHER ONE-DISH MEALS

Six-Layer Dinner

🌿

1½ pounds lean ground beef

4 medium potatoes, peeled and sliced thinly

2 large carrots, scraped and sliced

1 large onion, sliced thinly

1 medium green pepper (seeds removed), sliced

16-ounce can tomatoes, drained and chopped

½ teaspoon black pepper

⅛ teaspoon basil

Preheat over to 350°. In a large ovenproof pan with lid, brown ground beef over medium heat, stirring until crumbly. Drain well. Wipe pan with a paper towel to absorb grease. Return meat to pan and layer potatoes, carrots, onion, green pepper, and tomatoes over the top (in the order given). Do not stir. Sprinkle with pepper and basil. Cover with ovenproof lid and bake at 350° for 1 hour. Serve hot.

YIELD: 6 CUPS; 8 SERVINGS   4 G FAT   28 MG CHOLESTEROL
SERVING SIZE: ¾ CUP   1 G FIBER
CALORIES: 147   10 G PROTEIN
                             16 G CARBOHYDRATES

Ground Beef Pie Casserole

1½ pounds lean ground beef

¼ cup chopped onions

¼ cup chopped celery

2 tablespoons chopped green pepper

10¾-ounce can tomato soup

14¾-ounce can French-cut green beans

½ teaspoon black pepper

5 potatoes

¼ cup low-fat (2 percent) milk

2 tablespoons "lite" margarine

1. In a large skillet, brown ground beef with onion, celery, and green pepper. Add tomato soup and stir well. Pour mixture into a 9-by-13-inch baking pan. Stir in the green beans and black pepper.
2. Peel the potatoes and boil until soft. Mash with the milk and margarine.
3. Preheat oven to 350°. Place mounds of the mashed potatoes on top of meat and green bean mixture. Bake at 350° for 45 minutes or until potatoes are brown on top.

YIELD: 6 SERVINGS   8 G FAT   190 MG SODIUM
SERVING SIZE: ¾ CUP   5 G PROTEIN   8 MG CHOLESTEROL
CALORIES: 310   9 G CARBOHYDRATES

Chicken Broccoli Casserole

1 pound package frozen broccoli pieces

1½ pounds boneless, skinless chicken breasts, cut up

10¾-ounce can cream of mushroom soup, condensed

4-ounce can cream of broccoli soup

¼ cup water

4-ounce low-fat cheddar cheese, shredded

6-ounce package seasoned stuffing mix

Preheat oven to 350°. Place frozen broccoli in a 9-by-13-inch baking dish. Place chicken breasts on top of broccoli. Mix soups together with ¼ cup water and pour over the mixture. Sprinkle cheddar cheese on top, then sprinkle with the stuffing mix. Cover with foil. Bake at 350° for 1½ hours.

YIELD: 8 SERVINGS   7 G FAT   85 MG CHOLESTEROL
SERVING SIZE: ¾ CUP
CALORIES: 336

Chinese Noodle Casserole

❦

2½ to 3 cups cut-up cooked chicken

3-ounce can chow mein noodles

½ cup chopped celery

¼ cup minced onion

10¾-ounce can cream of celery soup, condensed

½ cup low-fat (2 percent) milk

4-ounce can mushroom pieces

1 cup chicken broth

Preheat oven to 350°. In a large bowl, mix the chicken, ¾ of the can of chow mein noodles, celery, onion, cream of celery soup, milk, mushrooms, and broth until well mixed. Pour into a 9-by-13-inch baking pan, cover, and bake at 350° for 30 minutes. Remove from oven, top with the remaining chow mein noodles. Return to oven, uncovered, and bake for 10 more minutes.

YIELD: 8 SERVINGS
SERVING SIZE: ¾ CUP
CALORIES: 260
EXCHANGES: 1½ STARCH/BREAD; 2 MEAT; 1 VEGETABLE; 1½ FAT

Ham-Topped Potatoes

4 medium baking potatoes

3 tablespoons cornstarch

2 cups low-fat (2 percent) milk

1 tablespoon Dijon mustard

¼ teaspoon pepper

½ cup shredded cheese, such as cheddar

10-ounce package frozen asparagus (or broccoli),
thawed and drained

2 cups chopped, fully cooked, extra-lean ham (8 ounces)

1. Arrange potatoes about 2 inches apart in microwave oven. Microwave on high for about 5 minutes. Turn, then microwave 5 more minutes, or until tender.

2. Mix cornstarch and milk in a 2-quart microwavable casserole. Microwave uncovered on high for 5 to 6 minutes, stirring every minute, until thickened. Stir in mustard, pepper, and cheese until cheese is melted. Stir in ham and asparagus or broccoli.

3. Peel potatoes and mash slightly. Place in a casserole and top with ham mixture. Microwave uncovered on high for 4 to 6 minutes or until heated through. (*Note:* The potatoes may be kept in their skins and the mixture poured over the potatoes, if desired.)

YIELD: 4 SERVINGS   5 G FAT   670 MG SODIUM

SERVING SIZE: ¾ CUP   75 MG CHOLESTEROL

CALORIES: 220

Low-Calorie Lasagna

1¼ pounds ground turkey

2 15-ounce cans tomato puree

2 cups water

½ cup chopped onion

½ cup chopped green pepper

⅛ teaspoon garlic powder

⅛ teaspoon oregano

1 tablespoon Italian dressing

nonstick vegetable spray

8-ounce package lasagna or regular noodles (uncooked)

8 ounces mozzarella cheese, grated or shredded

mushrooms (optional)

1.In a large skillet, brown the ground turkey. Combine the tomato puree, water, onion, green pepper, garlic powder, oregano, and Italian dressing with the turkey. Simmer for 15 minutes.

2.Preheat oven to 350°. Spray a 9-by-13-inch baking pan with nonstick cooking spray. Place ½ of the turkey and ½ of the sauce in the bottom of the pan. Layer noodles on top, then cover with the remaining turkey, mushrooms (optional), and sauce. Sprinkle with cheese. Cover and bake at 350° for 45 minutes or until lasagna is bubbly.

YIELD: 8 SERVINGS
SERVING SIZE: 1 3-BY-4-INCH SLICE
CALORIES: 150
EXCHANGES: 1 STARCH/BREAD; 3 MEAT; 1½ VEGETABLE

Potato-Crust Pizza

❦

8-ounce package frozen hash brown potatoes

4 ounces lean ground beef

4 ounces Italian or pork sausage

2 ounces pepperoni, sliced

2 ounces lean bacon, browned in microwave

2 tablespoons chopped onion

2 tablespoons chopped green peppers

2 tablespoons chopped celery

8 ounces mozzarella cheese, grated or shredded

1. Preheat oven to 350°. In a 12-inch deep-dish pizza pan, spread the hash brown potatoes and bake at 350° for 10 minutes. Remove from oven.
2. In a skillet, brown the ground beef and sausage. Drain well. Place on top of the potatoes. Next, place the pepperoni and bacon on top. Top with the onion, green pepper, and celery. Sprinkle cheese on top of the vegetables. Return to oven and bake for 15 to 20 minutes longer or until the cheese is melted and the vegetables are tender.

YIELD: 6 SERVINGS
SERVING SIZE: 1½ SLICES
CALORIES: 250
EXCHANGES: 3 STARCH/BREAD; 2 MEDIUM-FAT MEAT; 2 FAT

Vegetable Pizza

❧

8-roll package refrigerated crescent roll dough
8 ounces low-fat cream cheese
0.4-ounce package dry ranch dressing
¼ cup low-fat mayonnaise
2 tablespoons low-fat (2 percent) milk
½ cup chopped green pepper
½ cup chopped celery
¼ cup chopped onion
2 tomatoes, chopped
½ cucumber, thinly sliced

1. Preheat oven to 350°. Place dough on a nonstick cookie sheet and flatten to fill bottom of sheet. Bake 10 minutes at 350° or until golden brown. Remove from oven and let cool.
2. Combine cream cheese, ranch dressing, mayonnaise, and milk. Spread crust with this mixture. Top with layers of vegetables. Cut into small pieces and serve.

YIELD: 40 SMALL PIECES
SERVING SIZE: 2 PIECES
CALORIES: 145
EXCHANGES: ¼ STARCH/BREAD; ¼ VEGETABLE; ½ FAT

Hearty Tuna Casserole

2 (6.5-ounce) cans water-packed tuna
6 ounces uncooked egg noodles
½ cup chopped celery
⅓ cup chopped green onions
⅔ cup "lite" sour cream
½ cup low-fat mayonnaise
3 teaspoons prepared mustard
½ teaspoon thyme
¼ teaspoon salt
1 cup shredded Monterey Jack cheese
1 medium tomato, chopped

1. Drain and flake the tuna and set aside.
2. Cook the noodles according to the package directions. Drain and rinse in hot water.
3. Preheat oven to 350°. Combine the noodles with the tuna, celery, and green onions. Blend in the sour cream, mayonnaise, mustard, thyme, and salt. Spoon the mixture into a 2-quart casserole. Top with the cheese. Bake at 350° for 30 minutes, or until hot and bubbly. Sprinkle with chopped tomato.

YIELD: 5 SERVINGS   15 G FAT
SERVING SIZE: 1 CUP   18 G PROTEIN
CALORIES: 350   20 G CARBOHYDRATES

Wild Rice Casserole

❧

1 cup raw wild rice

nonstick vegetable spray

½ cup chopped onion

½ cup chopped celery

2 tablespoons chopped green pepper

1 clove chopped garlic

¼ cup chopped pecans

2½ cups chicken broth, preferably low-fat and reduced-sodium

¼ teaspoon black pepper

Prepare rice per package directions. Turn off the heat, wash rice, and let stand in the water until softened. Preheat oven to 325°. Spray a skillet and a 1½-quart casserole dish with nonstick vegetable spray. Sauté all vegetables in the sprayed skillet for 5 minutes or until soft. Add pecans and cook for 1 minute. Drain rice and add to vegetable mixture. Add chicken broth and pepper. Pour into prepared casserole dish. Cover and bake at 325° for 20 minutes.

YIELD: 8 SERVINGS
SERVING SIZE: ½ CUP
CALORIES: 128

3 G FAT
3 G FIBER
7 G PROTEIN
18 G CARBOHYDRATES

500 MG SODIUM
248 MG POTASSIUM
1 MG CHOLESTEROL

Crustless Zucchini Quiche

❦

½ cup chopped onion

1 teaspoon margarine

2 cups zucchini slices (¼ inch thick)

2 eggs

½ cup evaporated skim milk

½ teaspoon salt

⅛ teaspoon black pepper

dash of nutmeg

dash of paprika

½ cup Monterey Jack cheese, shredded

Preheat oven to 350°. Sauté onion in margarine for 2 to 3 minutes. Add zucchini and sauté for 5 more minutes. Beat eggs with milk and seasonings. Place zucchini mixture in an 8-inch glass pie plate. Pour egg mixture over zucchini and top with cheese. Bake at 350° for 45 minutes or until edges are brown and eggs are set. Cut into 4 wedges and serve.

YIELD: 4 SERVINGS	8 G FAT	425 MG SODIUM
SERVING SIZE: ¼ PIE	3 G FIBER	342 MG POTASSIUM
CALORIES: 142	2.4 G PROTEIN	152 MG CHOLESTEROL
	7 G CARBOHYDRATES	

Oven Baked Omelet

4 slices lean bacon

nonstick vegetable spray

3 slices processed low-fat American cheese

6 eggs, or 1½ cups egg substitute

¾ cup skim milk

¼ teaspoon salt

dash of pepper

Preheat oven to 350°. Cook bacon until crisp. Drain off fat and crumble bacon. Spray an 8-inch pie pan with nonstick vegetable spray. Arrange cheese slices in bottom of pan. Beat together eggs, milk, salt, and pepper; add bacon. Pour mixture over cheese. Bake at 350° for 30 minutes. Cut into 4 wedges and serve.

YIELD: 4 SERVINGS   10.2 G FAT   665.9 MG SODIUM
SERVING SIZE: 17.3 G PROTEIN   239.1 MG POTASSIUM
¼ OMELET   3.4 G CARBOHYDRATES 437 MG CHOLESTEROL
CALORIES: 250

Egg Substitute

❦

6 egg whites
¼ cup nonfat dry milk powder
1 tablespoon cooking oil
6 drops yellow food coloring
¾ cup water

Beat egg whites until stiff. Add powdered milk and oil. Beat well. Add food coloring and water. Mix well. This freezes well in ice cube trays.

YIELD: ¼ CUP (EQUIVALENT TO 1 EGG)
CALORIES: 50

Southwest Spanish Rice Casserole

6-ounce package Spanish rice mix

1½ pounds lean ground beef

1 small onion, chopped

¼ cup chopped celery

¼ cup chopped green pepper

1 teaspoon chili powder

14-ounce can stewed tomatoes

14-ounce can whole-kernel corn

¼ teaspoon salt (optional)

⅛ teaspoon black pepper

1. Prepare Spanish rice according to package directions.
2. In a frying pan, brown ground beef, onion, celery, pepper, and chili powder.
3. Preheat oven to 350°. In a casserole, mix the ground beef and rice mixture. Add the stewed tomatoes and corn. Season with salt and pepper. Bake at 350° for 1 hour.

YIELD: 8 SERVINGS
SERVING SIZE: ¾ CUP
CALORIES: 240
EXCHANGES: 1 STARCH/BREAD; 1 MEAT; 2 VEGETABLE

CAKES AND COOKIES

Danish Apple Cake

❧

When I was growing up, we always had this dessert (called *Aeblekage* in Danish) for Christmas Eve with real whipped cream on top; it was a special treat. Of course, now I substitute low-fat whipped topping; it's still delicious. My dad never wanted a birthday cake; he wanted this dessert instead. When my younger daughter was a little girl, she always wanted what her grandfather had.

Applesauce
5 large apples, such as Ida red or Cortland
½ cup water
½ teaspoon cinnamon
¼ teaspoon nutmeg
8 teaspoons sugar substitute or to taste,
depending on the sweetness of the apples

Cake
2 cups fine, very dry bread crumbs, made from leftover bread
½ cup "lite" margarine
3 cups thick applesauce
"lite" whipped topping (optional)

Peel apples and cut into small cubes. Put apple cubes in sauce pan; add water. Simmer uncovered for 10 minutes, stirring occasionally. Remove from stove; add cinnamon and nutmeg. Sweeten to taste. Stir well. Cover and let stand for about 30 minutes. Applesauce will be chunky.

Toast the bread crumbs in a 200° oven with the margarine—watch them closely, as they burn easily. Grease a 2-quart bowl. Place a layer of ½ cup bread crumbs on the bottom, next a layer of applesauce, and repeat until all is used, ending with crumbs. Cover and chill overnight. Serve with whipped topping (optional). (*Note:* This may also be baked in a slow oven [300°] for 1 hour. I like it best without baking.)

YIELD: 10 SERVINGS
SERVING SIZE: ½ CUP
CALORIES: 120

2 G FIBER
15 G CARBOHYDRATES

Banana Raspberry Layer Cake

½ cup evaporated skim milk, chilled

*10-ounce package fresh or defrosted frozen raspberries, drained;
reserve the juice*

1 envelope unflavored gelatin

¼ cup cold water

1 angel food cake, about 8 inches in diameter

2 ripe bananas, thinly sliced

fresh raspberries for garnish (optional)

1. Pour milk into ice cube tray and freeze until ice crystals begin to form around the edges.
2. Measure reserved raspberry juice and add enough water to make 1 cup. In a saucepan, combine gelatin with ¼ cup cold water to soften. Wait one minute, then heat gently until gelatin dissolves. Stir in reserved juice and refrigerate until cool.
3. In mixing bowl, combine chilled gelatin mixture with milk and beat until peaks form. Fold in berries.
4. Slice angel food cake horizontally into 3 layers. Frost first layer with ½ of berry mixture, top with ½ of the banana slices, add second cake layer, and top with remaining banana slices. Add third cake layer and spread top of cake with remaining raspberry mixture. Garnish with fresh raspberries, if desired. Chill thoroughly.

YIELD: 16 SERVINGS   0.2 G FAT   67.5 MG SODIUM
SERVING SIZE: 1 SLICE   3.6 G PROTEIN   0.3 MG CHOLESTEROL
CALORIES: 133   30.1 G CARBOHYDRATES

Easy Refrigerated Cheesecake

1 large package (8 servings) sugar-free gelatin, any flavor
2 cups hot water
1 cup cold water
4 ounces low-fat cream cheese, softened
8-ounce tub "lite" whipped topping
½ cup crushed graham crackers

Mix gelatin with hot water, stirring until dissolved, then add cold water. Chill until jellylike, but not firm. Beat in the softened cream cheese and the whipped topping. Sprinkle with crushed graham cracker crumbs. Refrigerate in an 8-inch square pan until firm, at least 2 hours.

YIELD: 6 SERVINGS
SERVING SIZE: ¼ CUP
CALORIES: 165
EXCHANGES: 1 FRUIT; 1 FAT

Old-Fashioned Lemon Cake

❦

This lemon cake is moist and dense, similar to pound cake.

nonstick vegetable spray

6 tablespoons "lite" margarine

8 packets sugar substitute (not Aspartame),
plus 2 tablespoons sugar

dash of salt

2 eggs

1½ cups flour

1 teaspoon baking powder

3 tablespoons lemon juice

1 teaspoon grated lemon peel

½ cup low-fat (2 percent) milk

Preheat oven to 325°. Spray a 9-by-5-inch loaf pan with nonstick vegetable spray. Cream margarine, sugar substitute, sugar, and salt together. Add eggs and beat well. Add flour, baking powder, lemon juice, lemon peel, and milk and beat well. Pour into prepared pan. Bake at 325° for 1 hour or until cake tester inserted in middle comes out clean. Cool on rack.

YIELD: 12 SLICES
SERVING SIZE: ½ SLICE
CALORIES: 138

7 G FAT
1 G FIBER
3 G PROTEIN
16 G CARBOHYDRATES

54 MG SODIUM
45 MG POTASSIUM
45 MG CHOLESTEROL

Pineapple Cheat Cake

20-ounce can crushed pineapple in its own juice, no sugar added
½ cup skimmed milk
1 envelope unflavored gelatin
8 ounces low-fat cream cheese
¼ teaspoon lemon juice
1 teaspoon vanilla extract
2 egg whites
12 packets sugar substitute

1. Drain pineapple and reserve the juice. If necessary, add water to juice to make 1 cup.

2. In a saucepan, mix milk and gelatin. Cook over low heat for 2 minutes, stirring constantly to dissolve gelatin completely. Remove from heat.

3. In a large bowl, beat cream cheese until smooth and fluffy. Gradually beat in hot gelatin/milk mixture and blend well. Next beat in pineapple juice, lemon juice, and vanilla. Chill until mixture holds a shape, about 30 to 35 minutes.

4. Beat egg whites until stiff and add sugar substitute. Fold egg whites and drained pineapple into cheese filling mixture. Turn into a 9-inch pan and chill until firm, about 4 to 5 hours.

YIELD: 8 SERVINGS
SERVING SIZE: 1 3-BY-3-INCH SQUARE
CALORIES: 114 CALORIES

5 G FAT
5 G PROTEIN
14 G CARBOHYDRATES

Easy Sugar-Free Shortcake

❦

These freeze very well. When fresh fruit is in season, I make a double batch and store them in the freezer to be used as needed. (Microwave on high 2 to 3 minutes to thaw and warm.) Topped with fresh fruit, these shortcakes make a dessert that's easy, healthy, and delicious. (Be sure to add the fruit exchanges to your daily intake tally.)

2 cups all-purpose baking mix
1 egg
⅔ cup low-fat (2 percent) milk

Preheat oven to 450°. Mix ingredients together until soft dough forms. Beat for 30 seconds. Drop by tablespoonfuls onto ungreased cookie sheet. Bake at 450° until golden brown, about 8 to 10 minutes.

YIELD: 10 BISCUITS
SERVING SIZE: 1 BISCUIT
CALORIES: 10
EXCHANGES: 1 STARCH/BREAD; ½ FAT

Easy Cheesecake

❦

1 cup graham cracker crumbs

¼ cup margarine, melted

32 ounces low-fat vanilla yogurt

3 tablespoons cornstarch

1 tablespoon sugar plus 1 tablespoon sugar substitute

1 teaspoon vanilla extract

2 eggs

1. Preheat oven to 425°. Mix together the graham cracker crumbs and the margarine. Press the mixture into the bottom of a 9-inch springform pan.

2. Combine the yogurt, cornstarch, sugar and sugar substitute, vanilla, and eggs in a bowl. Mix with a wire whisk until well blended. Pour the batter into the pan. Bake at 425° for 50 to 60 minutes or until the center is set. Cool and refrigerate until ready to serve.

YIELD: 12 SERVINGS

SERVING SIZE: 1-INCH

WEDGE

CALORIES: 175

6 G FAT

6 G PROTEIN

22 G CARBOHYDRATES

330 MG SODIUM

Chewy, Microwaved Coconut Bars

½ cup "lite" margarine

2 eggs

5 teaspoons sugar substitute

¼ teaspoon maple flavoring

1 teaspoon vanilla extract

1 cup flour

1 teaspoon baking powder

1 cup flaked coconut

½ cup chopped walnuts

½ cup raisins

Topping

1 teaspoon sugar substitute

1 teaspoon vanilla extract

8 maraschino cherries, sliced

1. Place margarine in a glass container and microwave for about 20 seconds on high until melted.
2. Beat eggs in a large bowl until light and fluffy. Add the sugar substitute, maple flavoring and vanilla, flour, baking powder, and melted margarine and blend thoroughly. Stir in coconut, nuts, and raisins.
3. Pour into an 8-inch square microwave-safe dish and microwave on high for 6 to 10 minutes: turn after 6 minutes, bake for another 4 minutes. Sprinkle with 1 teaspoon sugar substitute mixed with 1 teaspoon vanilla.

4. Let cool completely and then top with maraschino cherries. Cut into 24 bars.

YIELD: 24 BARS
SERVING SIZE: 1 BAR
CALORIES: 75
EXCHANGES: ½ STARCH/BREAD; 1 FAT

Rice Krispies™ Bars

¼ cup margarine
4 cups miniature marshmallows
6 cups Rice Krispies™

Melt margarine in a large pan over low heat. Add marshmallows and stir until completely melted. Remove from heat and add Rice Krispies™ and stir until they are coated and well mixed. Grease a 9-by-13-inch pan with margarine. Press mixture into pan. Cool. Cut into bars.

YIELD: 30 BARS
SERVING SIZE: 1 BAR
CALORIES: 65
EXCHANGES: ½ STARCH/BREAD   8 G CARBOHYDRATES

Snickerdoodles

1 cup "lite" margarine

6 packets sugar substitute, preferably acesulfame K

¼ cup sugar

2 eggs

1 teaspoon vanilla extract

2¼ cups flour

1 teaspoon baking soda

2 teaspoon cream of tartar

Cinnamon/sugar mixture: 2 tablespoons sugar
mixed with 2 teaspoons cinnamon

1. Preheat oven to 400°. Cream the margarine until light. Add the sugar substitute and sugar and beat until creamy. Add the eggs and vanilla and mix well.

2. Sift together the flour, baking soda, and cream of tartar. Add to margarine mixture and mix well.

3. Combine the sugar and cinnamon in a separate bowl. Put some flour on your hands to prevent the dough from sticking, and form the dough into small balls, about 1 inch in diameter, and roll in the cinnamon sugar mixture. Place on an ungreased cookie sheet, slightly apart (they will flatten out while baking) and bake at 400° for 8 to 10 minutes.

YIELD: 6 DOZEN COOKIES   17 MG SODIUM
CALORIES: 45 PER COOKIE   7.5 MG CHOLESTEROL

Rolled Sugar Cookies

½ cup "lite" margarine

¼ cup sugar

4 packets sugar substitute, preferably acesulfame K

1 egg

1 teaspoon vanilla extract

2 cups flour

2 teaspoons baking powder

1. Cream together margarine, sugar, sugar substitute, egg, and vanilla until well blended. Add the flour and baking powder. Blend until well mixed. Chill dough for 2 hours or overnight.

2. Preheat oven to 375°. Roll out dough on a lightly floured board until ⅛ inch thick, and cut with a cookie cutter. Place on an ungreased cookie sheet and bake at 375° for 9 to 10 minutes until lightly browned.

YIELD: 3 DOZEN COOKIES
CALORIES: 40 PER COOKIE

Oatmeal Cookies

1½ cups quick-cooking oatmeal, uncooked

⅔ cup "lite" margarine, melted

½ cup egg substitute

⅓ cup sugar

*sugar substitute equivalent to 1 cup plus 2 tablespoons sugar,
preferably acesulfame K*

1½ cups flour

½ teaspoon salt

2 teaspoons baking powder

½ teaspoon nutmeg

½ cup low-fat (2 percent) milk

1 teaspoon vanilla extract

¼ cup raisins

1. Measure oatmeal into a bowl. Stir in margarine and mix well. Stir in egg substitute, sugar, and sugar substitute. Add flour, salt, baking powder, and nutmeg alternately with milk. Add vanilla and raisins. Beat well.
2. Preheat oven to 350°. Drop by teaspoonfuls on a lightly greased cookie sheet. Bake at 350° for 12 minutes or until golden brown.

YIELD: 5 DOZEN COOKIES
CALORIES: 63 PER COOKIE
EXCHANGES: ¼ FRUIT; ¼ STARCH/BREAD; ¼ FAT

Grandma's Peanut Butter Cookies

❦

1 cup "lite" margarine

¾ cup brown sugar (or ¼ cup plus sugar substitute
equivalent to ½ cup)

¾ cup white sugar (or ¼ cup plus sugar substitute
equivalent to ½ cup)

2 eggs, beaten

1 teaspoon vanilla extract

1 cup peanut butter, creamy or chunky

1¼ cups flour

1 cup bran cereal (uncooked bran buds)

¾ cup quick-cooking oatmeal, uncooked

2 teaspoons baking soda

1. Melt margarine. Add sugars or sugar substitute, eggs, vanilla,
   and peanut butter and mix well.
2. In a separate bowl, combine flour, bran, oats, and baking soda.
   Stir this mixture into the margarine mixture. Blend well.
3. Preheat oven to 350°. Drop dough by teaspoonfuls on an ungreased cookie sheet. Flatten with a fork. Bake at 350° for 15
   to 18 minutes. Remove to a rack to cool.

YIELD: 7 DOZEN COOKIES   5.2 G FAT   75 MG SODIUM
SERVING SIZE: 2 COOKIES   1.9 G PROTEIN
CALORIES: 75 PER 2 COOKIES   7.2 G CARBOHYDRATES
IF SUGAR SUBSTITUTE IS USED

Peanut Butter Balls

½ cup unsweetened apple juice concentrate, thawed

⅔ cup peanut butter

3 tablespoons margarine

½ cup nonfat dry milk

3 cups bran cereal (uncooked bran buds)

In a saucepan, combine apple juice concentrate, peanut butter, and margarine and cook over low heat until melted. Bring to a boil, stirring constantly for 2 minutes. Remove from heat. Add milk and cereal. Roll into 1-inch balls or spoon into small mounds on waxed paper. Cool and store in a tightly covered container.

YIELD: 50 BALLS   4 G FAT   144 MG SODIUM
SERVING SIZE: 2 BALLS   4 G PROTEIN
CALORIES: 50   10 G CARBOHYDRATES

Lemon Cookies

1½ cups flour

1 tablespoon sugar

4 packets sugar substitute, preferably acesulfame K

¼ cup lemon juice

½ teaspoon grated lemon peel

6 tablespoons margarine

1 egg

nonstick vegetable spray

1 egg white, beaten lightly

1. In a mixing bowl, combine all ingredients, except egg white, and mix well. Flatten dough slightly. Cover with plastic wrap and chill for 30 minutes.

2. Break off a piece of dough and roll between your hands to form a rope. Make into a wreath or other desired shape.

3. Preheat oven to 350°. Spray a cookie sheet with nonstick vegetable spray. Place cookies on cookie sheet. Brush tops with egg white. Bake at 350° for 10 to 12 minutes or until golden brown.

YIELD: 30 COOKIES
SERVING SIZE: 2 COOKIES
CALORIES: 130
EXCHANGES: 1 STARCH/BREAD; 1 FAT

Mock Shortbread Cookies

2 cups all-purpose flour

1½ teaspoons baking powder

2 packets sugar substitute, preferably acesulfame K

½ cup cooking oil

¼ cup water

1 egg

1 teaspoon vanilla extract

nonstick vegetable spray

Preheat oven to 350°. Combine all ingredients to form a soft dough. Spray cookie sheet with nonstick vegetable spray. Roll or pat dough out on floured board to ¼ inch thick. Cut into 2-inch rounds and place 1 inch apart on cookie sheet. Bake at 350° for 15 to 20 minutes, or until edges are a light golden brown.

YIELD: 2 DOZEN COOKIES   5 G FAT   23 MG SODIUM
CALORIES: 89 PER COOKIE   1 G FIBER   14 MG POTASSIUM
                          2 G PROTEIN   11 MG CHOLESTEROL
                          9 G CARBOHYDRATES

Sugarless Cookies

1¾ cups flour

2 teaspoons baking powder

½ teaspoon salt

½ teaspoon cinnamon

1 egg

¾ cup unsweetened orange juice

½ cup (scant) cooking oil

½ teaspoon grated orange rind

½ cup raisins

½ cup chopped walnuts

Preheat oven to 375°. Combine flour, baking powder, salt, and cinnamon. Add egg, orange juice, oil, and orange rind. Mix well. Stir in raisins and nuts. Drop dough by teaspoonfuls on ungreased cookie sheet. Bake about 15 to 20 minutes. Remove from pan and cool.

YIELD: 32 TO 34 COOKIES

SERVING SIZE: 2 COOKIES

CALORIES: 161

EXCHANGES: 1 STARCH/ BREAD; ½ FAT

9.4 G FAT

1 G FIBER

2.7 G PROTEIN

17.1 G CARBOHYDRATES

111 MG SODIUM

93.8 MG POTASSIUM

17 MG CHOLESTEROL

Spice Cookies

❦

¼ teaspoon cooking oil

3 tablespoons diet margarine

1 tablespoon low-fat (2 percent) milk

1 egg

½ teaspoon vanilla extract

1½ cups white flour

1 teaspoon baking powder

½ teaspoon cinnamon

½ teaspoon nutmeg

½ teaspoon ginger

½ teaspoon cloves

Glaze

2 teaspoons sugar substitute

½ teaspoon cinnamon

2 tablespoons hot water

Preheat oven to 375°. In a mixing bowl, beat together oil and margarine. Add milk, egg, and vanilla and blend well. Combine dry ingredients and blend into liquids. Roll into 1-inch balls and flatten balls with the tines of a fork. Place on a nonstick cookie sheet 2 inches apart. Bake at 375° for 8 to 10 minutes. Combine glaze mixture and brush onto cookies.

YIELD: 24 COOKIES
SERVING SIZE: 2 COOKIES
CALORIES: 100
EXCHANGES: 1 STARCH/BREAD; 1 FAT

DESSERTS

Baked Custard

3 eggs, lightly beaten

2 tablespoons sugar

¼ teaspoon salt

⅛ teaspoon nutmeg

2 cups skim milk

½ teaspoon vanilla extract

dash of cinnamon

Preheat oven to 325°. Combine eggs, sugar, salt, and nutmeg. Slowly stir in milk and vanilla. Set 6 custard cups in shallow pan. Pour hot water in pan to level of about 1 inch. Pour custard into cups. Sprinkle with cinnamon. Bake at 325° for 40 minutes or until knife inserted in center comes out clean.

YIELD: 6 SERVINGS, 3 CUPS
SERVING SIZE: ½ CUP
CALORIES: 83
2.9 G FAT
5.8 G PROTEIN
8.2 G CARBOHYDRATES
165.3 MG SODIUM
167.8 MG POTASSIUM
138 MG CHOLESTEROL

Rhubarb Dessert

This recipe took some experimenting. It's based on a Danish dish called *Rabarbergrod*. We like rhubarb, so I kept working at it. I use it as an upside-down cake.

2 ounces rhubarb, cut up into 1-inch pieces (about 2½ cups)
1 small package (4 servings) sugar-free strawberry gelatin
2 tablespoons sugar
3 packets sugar substitute
1 package sugar-free white cake mix
"lite" frozen whipped topping, thawed (optional)

Preheat oven to 375°. Lightly oil an 8-inch square pan. Mix rhubarb, gelatin, sugar, and sugar substitute together. Place in bottom of pan. Prepare cake mix as directed on box. Pour over rhubarb mixture. Bake at 375° for 30 minutes or until tester comes out clean. Top with whipped topping if desired.

YIELD: 9 SERVINGS
SERVING SIZE: ⅑ OF RECIPE
CALORIES: 115 (ADD CALORIES IF TOPPING USED)
EXCHANGES: 1 FRUIT; 1 STARCH/BREAD; 1 FAT

Berry Dips

❦

2 cups "lite" frozen whipped topping, thawed
1 tablespoon grated orange peel;
or 2 tablespoons unsweetened orange juice
½ cup crushed strawberries
1 cup low-fat strawberry yogurt
fresh strawberries, peach slices, or melon slices
pound cake or angel food cake, cubed

Mix ½ of the whipped topping and orange peel together. Mix remaining whipped topping, strawberries, and yogurt in a separate bowl. Dip whole strawberries, cake cubes, peach slices, and melon slices into mixture.

YIELD: 5¼ CUPS; 20 SERVINGS
SERVING SIZE: ¼ CUP DIP AND 2-BY-2-INCH SLICE OF FRUIT OR CAKE
CALORIES: 40 FOR CAKE (DIP VARIES BY KIND OF FRUIT USED)
EXCHANGES: 3 FRUIT; 2 FAT

Fruity Ice Milk

❦

1 cup "lite" frozen whipped topping, thawed
1 egg, separated
3 packets sugar substitute
1 teaspoon vanilla extract
1 cup fresh fruit (strawberries, peaches, blueberries, or raspberries)

Thaw whipped topping and fold in egg yolk and sugar substitute. In a separate bowl, beat egg white until stiff peaks form, and add vanilla. Gently fold egg white into whipped topping. Freeze for 30 minutes, then beat again. Fold in fresh fruit. Pour mixture into a refrigerator tray or 6 foil-lined muffin cups. Freeze until firm.

YIELD: 6 SERVINGS   1 G FAT   2 MG SODIUM
SERVING SIZE: ¼ CUP   3 G CARBOHYDRATES
CALORIES: 24
EXCHANGES: UP TO ¼ CUP
IS A FREE FOOD

Fresh Fruit Bavarian Cream

1 cup evaporated skim milk
1 large (8 servings) package sugar-free strawberry gelatin
1½ cups boiling water
1 graham cracker pie crust
1 cup sliced fresh strawberries or other fruit

1. Pour evaporated milk into an ice cube tray and freeze until crystals begin to form around edges.
2. Dissolve gelatin in boiling water.
3. Chill gelatin until syrupy. Beat the chilled milk at high speed until stiff, about 8 minutes. Gently fold milk into gelatin mixture until well blended.
4. Arrange fruit in bottom of pie crust. Pour filling on top of the fruit. Refrigerate several hours or overnight.

YIELD: 8 SERVINGS
SERVING SIZE: ⅛ OF RECIPE
CALORIES: 162

3.1 G FAT
5.1 G PROTEIN
30 G CARBOHYDRATES

1.3 MG CHOLESTEROL

Ambrosia Fruit Cocktail

1 banana, sliced

2 oranges, peeled, seeded, and cut into chunks

8-ounce can pineapple chunks, in its own juice, undrained

*2 tablespoons frozen unsweetened pineapple juice concentrate,
defrosted and undiluted*

4 teaspoons flaked coconut

Combine fruits and pineapple juice concentrate. Stir well and spoon into 4 glasses. Sprinkle with coconut. Chill and serve.

YIELD: 4 SERVINGS   0.6 G FAT   2.7 MG SODIUM
SERVING SIZE: APPROX. 1 CUP   1.1 G PROTEIN
CALORIES: 110   26.4 G CARBOHYDRATES

Banana Orange Gelatin

1 large banana
¼ cup cold water
1 small package (4 servings) sugar-free orange gelatin,
1 cup boiling water
16-ounce can unsweetened frozen orange juice concentrate

Slice banana into a bowl. Pour ¼ cup cold water into a mixing bowl and sprinkle gelatin on top. Stir. Add 1 cup boiling water and stir until gelatin is thoroughly dissolved. Add orange juice concentrate and mix well. Pour over banana slices. Chill until set.

YIELD: 4 SERVINGS   28.1 G CARBOHYDRATES   3.6 MG SODIUM
SERVING SIZE: APPROX.
½ CUP
CALORIES: 127

Strawberry Mousse

✿

1 small package (4 servings) sugar-free strawberry gelatin
¾ cup boiling water
1 cup ice cubes
1 cup strawberries, sliced
½ cup "lite" frozen whipped topping, thawed

Combine gelatin with boiling water, stirring well. Add ice cubes and stir again, until ice cubes are melted. Add sliced strawberries and blend well. Add whipped topping and stir until well mixed. Chill until set.

YIELD: 4 SERVINGS
SERVING SIZE: APPROX. ½ CUP
CALORIES: 50
EXCHANGES: ½ FRUIT; ½ FAT

Fruit Frappé

❧

1 small (4 servings) package sugar-free lime gelatin
¾ cup boiling water
2 cups ice cubes
½ cup lemon or lime sherbet

Pour ¾ boiling water into a blender. Add gelatin and blend at low speed until well dissolved. Add ice cubes and stir until partially melted, then blend until mixture is slightly thickened. Add sherbet and blend. Pour into dessert glasses and chill until set, approximately 1 hour, or serve immediately as a beverage.

YIELD: 5
SERVING SIZE: APPROX. ½ CUP
CALORIES: 35

Strawberry Frozen Dessert

❦

10-ounce package frozen strawberries, no sugar added

3 tablespoons frozen lemonade concentrate

6 tablespoons sugar or equivalent sugar substitute

1½ cups evaporated skim milk

1 egg white for meringue (optional)

9-inch meringue pie shell (optional),
or a prepared graham cracker crust

Combine frozen strawberries, lemonade, sugar, and milk in a blender and blend until smooth. Process in an ice cream maker until firm; or the mix may be frozen in a pie shell. If using a meringue pie shell, add 1 egg white, stiffly beaten, to the mixture.

YIELD: 9 SERVINGS   0 G FAT   55 MG SODIUM
SERVING SIZE: ½ CUP   4 G PROTEIN
CALORIES: 110   25 G CARBOHYDRATES
EXCHANGES: 2 FRUITS

Cool and Light Lime Dessert

✿

8-ounce can evaporated skim milk

1 small (4 servings) package sugar-free lime gelatin

1 tablespoon sugar

3 packets sugar substitute

¼ cup lemon juice

dash of white vinegar

*8-ounce can crushed pineapple in its own juice, drained;
reserve juice*

1 cup boiling water

1⅓ cups graham cracker crumbs

Chill evaporated milk in refrigerator overnight. The next day, stir together gelatin, sugar, sugar substitute, lemon juice, vinegar, reserved pineapple juice, and 1 cup boiling water until dissolved. Refrigerate until partially set. Beat until light and frothy. Beat chilled evaporated milk until peaks form. Fold into lime mixture with crushed pineapple. Line a 9-by-13-inch pan with 1 cup graham cracker crumbs. Pour in gelatin mixture and top with remaining crumbs. Chill well before serving.

YIELD: 12 SERVINGS   1 G FAT
SERVING SIZE: 3-BY-4-INCH PIECE
CALORIES: 95

Chilled Orange Soufflé

❦

1 envelope unflavored gelatin

¼ cup sugar

1 cup cold water

6-ounce can frozen unsweetened orange juice concentrate,
undiluted, thawed

½ cup ice water

½ cup instant nonfat dry milk crystals

2 tablespoons lemon juice

sugar substitute equivalent to ¼ cup sugar

1 cup nonfat frozen whipped topping, thawed

fresh fruit (cantaloupe, honeydew melon, green grapes, blueberries,
or other fresh fruit) for garnish

1. Mix together gelatin and ¼ cup sugar in a saucepan. Stir in 1
   cup cold water. Place over low heat, stirring constantly, until
   gelatin is dissolved. Remove from heat and stir in orange
   juice concentrate. Chill, stirring occasionally, until the mixture is the consistency of unbeaten egg whites.

2. While mixture is chilling, pour ½ cup of ice water into a mixing bowl and add nonfat dry milk crystals. Beat until soft
   peaks form, about 4 minutes. Add lemon juice and continue
   beating until firm peaks form, about 4 minutes longer. Gradually add the sugar substitute to the milk mixture, then fold
   into gelatin mixture. Turn into a mold or a glass bowl. Chill
   until firm. Garnish with whipped topping and fresh fruit.

YIELD: 8 SERVINGS   0.1 G FAT   23 MG SODIUM
SERVING SIZE: ⅛ OF MOLD   1.9 G PROTEIN   0.9 MG CHOLESTEROL
CALORIES: 110   25.8 G CARBOHYDRATES

Microwaved Fresh Fruit Crisp

※

½ cup quick-cooking rolled oats, uncooked

brown sugar substitute equal to ½ cup brown sugar

¼ cup flour

1 teaspoon cinnamon

dash of salt

¼ cup "lite" margarine

7 or 8 apples, peeled and sliced (about 4 cups)

In a mixing bowl, mix together the oats, sugar substitute, flour, cinnamon, and salt. Cut in margarine until mixture is crumbly. Set aside. Place the apple slices in an 8-inch square pan. Sprinkle with the oat mixture. Bake in a microwave oven on medium for 15 minutes or until fruit is done. (*Note:* Peaches, pears, or cherries may be substituted for the apples.)

YIELD: 6 SERVINGS
SERVING SIZE: 4 X 2¾-INCH PIECE
CALORIES: 175
EXCHANGES: 1½ FRUIT; ½ STARCH/BREAD

Pear Fluff

¼ cup unsweetened orange juice
1 tablespoon lemon juice
1 tablespoon tapioca granules
2 large pears, peeled, cored, and diced
2 egg whites
1 tablespoon unsweetened apple juice concentrate, thawed

1. Preheat oven to 425°. Mix orange juice, lemon juice, and tapioca in a saucepan. Add pears. Cook over medium heat until sauce thickens, stirring constantly. Pour into a greased 8-inch baking pan.
2. Beat egg whites until almost stiff. Add apple juice concentrate and continue beating until stiff. Pour egg whites over pear mixture and bake at 425° for 5 to 7 minutes or until golden brown. May be served warm or at room temperature.

YIELD: 4 SERVINGS
SERVING SIZE: 4-BY-4-INCH PIECE
CALORIES: 84

0.3 G FAT
2.0 G PROTEIN
18.5 G CARBOHYDRATES

Frozen Blueberry Creme

1 packet unflavored gelatin

¼ cup cold water

1 cup fresh blueberries, washed and stemmed

1½ cups evaporated skim milk

9 packets sugar substitute

1 tablespoon sugar

3 tablespoons lemon juice

1. Sprinkle gelatin over ¼ cup cold water in a saucepan.
2. Reserving a few whole berries for garnish, puree blueberries in blender with 1 cup of evaporated skim milk, sugar substitute, and sugar.
3. Dissolve gelatin over low heat and stir in lemon juice. Stir gelatin into blueberry mixture.
4. Whip remaining ½ cup evaporated milk until thick but not stiff. Fold into blueberry mixture. Pour into a 2-quart bowl. Freeze for several hours, stirring occasionally, until mushy. Spoon into dessert dishes while still soft. Garnish with reserved blueberries.

YIELD: 8 SERVINGS
SERVING SIZE: ½ CUP
CALORIES: 53
EXCHANGES: ½ SKIM MILK

0 G FAT
1 G FIBER
5 G PROTEIN
9 G CARBOHYDRATES

58 MG SODIUM
203 MG POTASSIUM
2 MG CHOLESTEROL

Fresh Fruit Dessert

1¾ cups low-fat (2 percent) milk
1 tablespoon unsweetened orange juice
1 small (4 servings) package sugar-free instant vanilla pudding mix
1 cup "lite" frozen whipped topping, thawed
6 cups fresh fruit such as strawberries, raspberries,
grapes, apples, or oranges

Pour milk and orange juice into a bowl; add pudding mix and beat slowly with a hand beater or an electric beater at lowest speed for 1 minute. Add whipped topping and beat 1 minute longer. Arrange half of the fruit in a large serving bowl. Top with the pudding mixture, then top with the remaining fruit.

YIELD: 10 SERVINGS
SERVING SIZE: ¾ CUP
CALORIES: 150
EXCHANGES: 3 FRUITS; 1 MILK; ½ FAT

Homemade Ice Cream

I had several snafus along the way developing this recipe. I had to guess estimate the amounts of sugar and sugar substitute; sometimes it was too sweet and at other times, not the right consistency. I tried several different flavors and combinations, too.

Some were great: plain strawberry, raspberry, chocolate, and pineapple. Some combinations worked fine on the first try, especially if I was just adding something like nuts to a flavor that was already a "keeper" (although I found out that almonds don't work with some fruits and other nuts). Other combinations with any flavor other than Hershey's syrup and vanilla were a disaster. Pineapple with coconut and nuts turned out stringy and tasted awful. But I finally got several variations down pat. It's a delicious and refreshing dish, equivalent to frozen yogurt or ice milk.

6 whole eggs
¾ cup sugar
sugar substitute equivalent to 1¼ cups sugar
14-ounce can low-fat sweetened condensed milk
4 teaspoons vanilla extract
½ teaspoon salt
1½ quarts low-fat (2 percent) milk

In a large bowl, beat eggs until frothy. Add the sugar and sugar substitute, condensed milk, vanilla, and salt and mix well. Add the low-fat milk and stir gently. Pour the mixture into an ice cream maker and follow directions for freezing. (If using fruit, nuts, or chocolate, add these before pouring into the ice cream maker.)

YIELD: 1 GALLON
SERVING SIZE: ½ CUP
CALORIES: 136 (FOR VANILLA ICE CREAM)
EXCHANGES: 1 STARCH/BREAD; 1 FAT

Snickers™ Dessert

❦

This dish was much too rich and sweet for me, so I had to modify it. It's still rather rich, but it's better for my diet now and is a nice treat occasionally.

*2 cups nonfat, sugar-free, vanilla or praline ice cream
or frozen yogurt*
1 cup "lite" sugar-free frozen whipped topping, thawed
¼ cup peanut butter
1 small (4 servings) package sugar-free butterscotch pudding mix

Mix all ingredients thoroughly and pour into an 8-inch square pan. Freeze.

YIELD: 8 SERVINGS
SERVING SIZE: 2-BY-2-INCH PIECE
CALORIES: 135 WHEN MADE WITH FROZEN YOGURT
EXCHANGES: 1 MILK; 2½ FAT

Fat-Free Strawberry Ice Milk

❦

2 teaspoons unflavored gelatin

1 cup cold water

¾ cup instant nonfat dry milk crystals

1½ cups skim milk

⅔ cup sugar (half of this can be replaced with equivalent
amount of sugar substitute)

2 teaspoons vanilla extract

1 tablespoon lemon juice

1 cup mashed fresh or frozen unsweetened strawberries

1. Soften the gelatin in ½ cup cold water. Combine ¼ cup of the milk crystals with the skim milk and heat slowly in a saucepan. Add the gelatin mixture and heat until dissolved. Stir in ½ cup of the sugar until dissolved. Stir in the vanilla. Chill until slightly thickened.

2. Beat the remaining ½ cup milk crystals with the remaining ½ cup of cold water until it begins to thicken slightly. Add the lemon juice and remaining sugar and beat for 5 minutes or until the consistency of whipped cream. Add the mashed strawberries, and fold in the chilled gelatin mixture. Spoon into refrigerator trays. Freeze until the edges are set.

3. Remove to mixer bowl and beat on high speed until fluffy. Cover and freeze until firm.

YIELD: 8 SERVINGS   0.7 G FAT   58 MG SODIUM
SERVING SIZE: ½ CUP   4.4 G PROTEIN   2.3 MG CHOLESTEROL
CALORIES: 116.5   24.6 G CARBOHYDRATES

Fresh Peach Sherbet Royal

✤

2 medium peaches, peeled and sliced
⅔ cup skim milk
⅔ cup diet lemon–lime soda
1 tablespoon peach schnapps (optional)
1 egg white
5 packets sugar substitute

Blend peaches, milk, and lemon-lime soda in a blender until smooth. Add peach schnapps, egg white, and sugar substitute. Blend until smooth. Freeze in pie plate until partially firm (1 to 1½ hours); break up with a fork or puree. Cover and freeze until firm.

YIELD: 5 SERVINGS 0 G FAT 30 MG SODIUM
(2½ CUPS) 1 G FIBER 167 MG POTASSIUM
SERVING SIZE: ½ CUP 2 G PROTEIN 1 MG CHOLESTEROL
CALORIES: 52 11 G CARBOHYDRATES
EXCHANGES: 1 FRUIT

Cherry Yogurt Jubilee

❦

1 quart low-fat vanilla frozen yogurt
16-ounce can pitted and chopped dark red cherries, in their own juice; or 1 quart fresh cherries may be used
2 teaspoons cornstarch
3 tablespoons brandy

Scoop yogurt into 8 sherbet glasses and place in freezer until serving time. Combine cherries and cornstarch in a chafing dish. Stir over moderate flame until sauce simmers and clears. Pour brandy into the sauce. Carefully ignite the vapors with a long match. Spoon flaming cherries over the yogurt and serve immediately.

YIELD: 8 SERVINGS   2.1 G FAT   5.5 MG CHOLESTEROL
SERVING SIZE: ½ CUP   4.0 G PROTEIN
CALORIES: 123   21.6 G CARBOHYDRATES

Pie Crust

❦

¾ cup oatmeal

¾ cup Grape-Nuts™ cereal

1 teaspoon cinnamon

¼ cup apple juice concentrate

Preheat oven at 350°. Mix oatmeal and Grape-Nuts™ in a food processor. Add cinnamon and apple juice concentrate. Press into pie plate. Bake at 350° for 10 minutes.

Key Lime Pie

❦

¼ cup sugar

6 packets sugar substitute

1 tablespoon cornstarch

⅓ cup lime juice

⅓ cup water

1 large egg yolk

1 teaspoon grated lime peel

1 envelope unflavored gelatin

1¼ cups skim milk

1 teaspoon vanilla extract

⅓ cup nonfat frozen whipped topping, thawed

1 prepared pie crust

fresh fruit for garnish (optional)

1. In top of a double boiler, combine sugar, 4 packets sugar substitute, and cornstarch. Whisk in lime juice, water, egg yolk, and lime peel until well blended. Cook over hot water, stirring constantly, for 5 minutes. Refrigerate for 30 minutes or until well chilled.
2. Sprinkle gelatin over ¼ cup milk to soften it. Cook over low heat stirring until gelatin dissolves. Pour into a large bowl. Add remaining milk, vanilla, and remaining 2 packets sugar substitute. Refrigerate until mixture begins to gel.
3. Beat chilled mixture until fluffy. Fold in whipped topping. Fold lime mixture into gelatin until well blended. Mix well. Spoon into prepared crust. Garnish with fresh fruit if desired.

YIELD: 8 SERVINGS
SERVING SIZE: ⅛ PIE
CALORIES: 120
EXCHANGE: 1 FRUIT; 1 STARCH/BREAD; 3 FAT

Lemon Pie

❧

1⅔ cups graham cracker crumbs

⅓ cup "lite" margarine, melted

¼ cup sugar (half of this can be replaced with the equivalent amount of sugar substitute)

1 envelope unflavored gelatin

½ cup cold water

8 ounces low-fat lemon yogurt

¾ cup nonfat mayonnaise

1 cup "lite" frozen whipped topping, thawed

fresh fruit for garnish (optional)

1. Preheat oven to 350°. Mix graham cracker crumbs, margarine, and sugar. Press into bottom and up the sides of a 9-inch pie pan. Bake 8 to 10 minutes at 350°. Cool.

2. Soften gelatin in ½ cup cold water in a saucepan, over low heat, stirring until dissolved. Beat yogurt and mayonnaise at medium speed with an electric mixer until well blended. Fold in thawed whipped topping. Pour into crust. Chill until firm. Garnish with fresh fruit if desired.

YIELD: 8 SERVINGS   6 G FAT   5 G CHOLESTEROL
SERVING SIZE: ⅛ PIE
CALORIES: 200

Impossible Pecan Date Pie

I like pecan pie. When I was first diagnosed with diabetes, I thought I would never be able to have it again. I decided to work on the recipe and see what I could do with it. The first attempt was a fiasco: too sweet, too rich. Another attempt was likewise inedible. Later, while my husband and I were vacationing in Arizona, I bought some fresh dates. It occurred to me then to try dates in the pecan pie recipe. I made it as a custard and was surprised and delighted that it made its own crust. This is not as sweet as a regular pecan pie, but it is a good substitute. It still has considerable fat and cholesterol, but it is a great treat occasionally.

1 cup chopped pecans
¼ cup flour
1 cup chopped dates
4 eggs
½ cup "lite" margarine, melted
1 cup skim milk
1 teaspoon vanilla extract

Preheat oven to 350°. Lightly grease a 9-inch pie pan. Sprinkle with pecans. In a blender, mix remaining ingredients until well blended. Pour over pecans. Bake at 350° until set, about 30 minutes. Custard is done when a knife inserted in center comes out clean.

YIELD: 12 SLICES   17 G FAT   93 MG CHOLESTEROL
SERVING SIZE: 1 SLICE   4.3 G PROTEIN
CALORIES: 230

Fresh Strawberry Pie

1½ cups water

1 tablespoon cornstarch

4 packages sugar substitute

1 small (4 servings) sugar-free package strawberry gelatin

4 cups sliced fresh strawberries

1 prepared pie crust

In a medium saucepan, mix water and cornstarch. Cook over medium heat until bubbles form, stirring constantly. Remove from heat, sprinkle sugar substitute and gelatin over mixture. Stir and let cool. Fold in strawberries and pour into crust.

YIELD: 8 SERVINGS
SERVING SIZE: ⅛ PIE
CALORIES: 110
EXCHANGES: 1 FRUIT; 1 STARCH/BREAD; 1 FAT

Fresh Blueberry Pie

4 cups fresh blueberries

2 tablespoons sugar substitute

1 tablespoon honey

1½ teaspoons cornstarch

*1 prepared pie crust (graham or shortbread is
very good with this filling)*

In a nonstick saucepan, combine 2 cups of the blueberries with sugar substitute, honey, and cornstarch. Simmer over low heat for 10 minutes, stirring occasionally, until berries are softened and slightly thickened. Remove from heat and stir in remaining berries. Allow to cool. Spoon into crust and chill thoroughly before serving.

YIELD: 8 SERVINGS
SERVING SIZE: ⅛ PIE
CALORIES: 140
EXCHANGES: 1 FRUIT; 1 FAT

Blueberry Yogurt Pie

16 ounces blueberry yogurt
1 cup "lite" frozen whipped topping, thawed
10-ounce package frozen blueberries (no sugar added),
thawed slightly
1 prepared pie crust

In a bowl, fold blueberry yogurt into the whipped topping. Fold the blueberries into the yogurt mixture. Pour into crust. Freeze for 3 to 4 hours. Remove from freezer about 20 minutes before serving.

YIELD: 8 SERVINGS
SERVING SIZE: ⅛ PIE
CALORIES: 160
EXCHANGES: 1 FRUIT; 1 STARCH/BREAD; 1½ FAT

Easy Sugar-Free
Banana Cream Pie

*1 small (4 servings) package sugar-free vanilla pudding mix
(not instant)*

2 cups low-fat (2 percent) milk

2 bananas

1 graham cracker crust

Prepare pudding with milk. Slice 1 banana into the bottom of the prepared crust. Slice other banana into the prepared pudding. Pour pudding into the crust. Chill.

YIELD: 6 SERVINGS
SERVING SIZE: ⅙ PIE
CALORIES: 205
EXCHANGES: 1 FRUIT; 1 STARCH/BREAD; 1½ FAT

Deep-Dish Pear Pie

When I was a little girl, we had guests from New Mexico; a World War I Army buddy of my dad's came with his wife and young son to spend a week with my family. My mother was planning to make apple pies for dessert one day. Since we had a pear tree in our yard and it was ripe with fruit at the time, our guest asked if she'd also make a pear pie. My mom had never heard of a pear pie, but as it was our guest's favorite pie, she said she would try. She made one apple pie and one pear pie—which turned out fine. In fact, I liked it so much, it became one of my favorites. When I became diabetic, the recipe had to be modified. After several tries and many modifications, my family likes this version as well as we did my mother's original recipe.

9-inch deep-dish pie crust (unbaked)

Filling

6 pears
2 tablespoons white flour
1 cup nonfat lemon yogurt
¼ teaspoon cinnamon
¼ cup sugar
sugar substitute equivalent to ¼ cup sugar
1 egg
⅛ teaspoon salt
1 teaspoon vanilla extract

Topping

3 tablespoons sugar substitute

½ teaspoon cinnamon

½ teaspoon nutmeg

4 teaspoons "lite" margarine

1. Preheat oven to 400°. Peel pears, core, and cut into bite-sized pieces. Set aside.
2. In a large bowl, combine remaining filling ingredients and fold into pears. Pour pear mixture into pie crust and bake at 400° for 10 minutes. Lower heat to 350° and continue baking for 30 to 35 minutes more.
3. Mix together topping ingredients. Remove pie from oven and sprinkle topping over filling. Raise heat to 375° and bake until topping is browned.

YIELD: 12 SLICES
SERVING SIZE: 1 SLICE
CALORIES: 210

7.4 G FAT (30% CALORIES FROM FAT)
148 MG SODIUM
18 MG CHOLESTEROL

Deep-Dish Apple Pie

9-inch deep-dish pie crust (unbaked)

Filling
6 apples

2 tablespoons white flour

1 cup nonfat plain yogurt

½ teaspoon cinnamon

¼ teaspoon nutmeg

2 tablespoons sugar

*sugar substitute equivalent to ¼ cup sugar,
preferably acesulfame K*

1 egg

⅛ teaspoon salt

1 teaspoon vanilla extract

Topping
3 tablespoons sugar substitute

½ teaspoon cinnamon

3 tablespoons white flour

4 teaspoons "lite" margarine

1. Preheat oven to 400°. Peel apples and cut into bite-sized pieces. Set aside.

2. In a large bowl, combine remaining filling ingredients and fold into apples. Pour apple mixture into pie crust and bake at 400° for 10 minutes. Lower heat to 350° and continue baking for 30 to 35 minutes more.

3. Mix together topping ingredients. Remove pie from oven and sprinkle topping over filling. Raise heat to 375° and bake until topping is browned.

YIELD: 12 SLICES
SERVING SIZE: 1 SLICE
CALORIES: 210

7.4 G FAT (30% CALORIES FROM FAT)
148 MG SODIUM
18 MG CHOLESTEROL

Pumpkin Chiffon Pie

❧

1 tablespoon unflavored gelatin

½ cup cold water

3 eggs, separated

½ cup low-fat (2 percent) milk

1¼ cups canned pumpkin

½ teaspoon salt

¾ teaspoon cinnamon

½ teaspoon nutmeg

½ teaspoon ginger

½ teaspoon allspice

sugar substitute to equal ½ cup sugar

2 tablespoons sugar

1 graham cracker crust

2 squares graham crackers, crushed, for garnish

1. Dissolve gelatin in ½ cup cold water; set aside.
2. Beat egg yolks lightly; stir in milk, pumpkin, salt, and spices. Blend well. Cook in the top of a double boiler, stirring constantly, until smooth and thick, 7 or 8 minutes. Remove from heat.
3. Add gelatin and artificial sweetener; stir until completely dissolved. Cool, then chill in refrigerator until mixture thickens.

4. Remove from refrigerator. Beat egg whites until soft peaks form. Add sugar gradually to egg whites, beating constantly until glossy and stiff. Fold carefully into pumpkin mixture and stir lightly. Pour carefully into the prepared pie crust and sprinkle with crushed graham crackers. Chill at least 8 hours.

YIELD: 8 SERVINGS
SERVING SIZE: ⅛ PIE
CALORIES: 165
EXCHANGES: 1 FRUIT; 2 FAT; 1 MEAT

Easy Fruit Juice Tapioca

🌱

2½ cups unsweetened pineapple juice
(or other unsweetened juice of your choice)
¼ cup quick-cooking tapioca
pinch of ground cinnamon or apple pie spice

Combine all ingredients in a saucepan. Wait 5 minutes so that items are well blended. Then cook and stir over low heat until mixture simmers and begins to boil. Remove from heat and cover. Wait 25 to 30 minutes, then stir well. Spoon into dessert dishes and chill for several hours.

YIELD: 6 SERVINGS   0 G FAT   1.0 MG SODIUM
SERVING SIZE: ¼ CUP   0.4 G PROTEIN
CALORIES: 78   19.6 G CARBOHYDRATES

Chilled Peach Soufflé

Other fruits, such as strawberries, raspberries, blueberries, or pears, can be substituted for the peaches.

16-ounce can sliced peaches in their own juice
1 packet unflavored gelatin
¼ cup boiling water
3 packets sugar substitute
1 egg, separated ½ cup skim milk
1½ teaspoons lemon juice
¼ cup ice cubes
1-ounce packet whipped topping mix
1 teaspoon vanilla extract

1. Drain peaches, reserving juice. Measure ¼ cup juice and set aside. Place remaining juice in blender, add gelatin and soften for 1 minute. Pour boiling water into blender and blend until frothy. Add all but 4 slices of the peaches (save those for garnish), sugar substitute, egg yolk, and lemon juice. Blend until smooth. Add ice cubes and blend until ice is melted. Pour mixture into a bowl and refrigerate.

2. Beat egg white until stiff and gently fold into the peach mixture. Whip topping mix with the skim milk and vanilla until stiff; then gently fold into the peach mixture. Turn into a soufflé dish and chill until firm. Keep refrigerated until serving. At serving time, garnish with reserved peach slices.

YIELD: 8 SERVINGS   2 G FAT   20 MG SODIUM
SERVING SIZE: ¼ CUP   1 G FIBER   130 MG POTASSIUM
CALORIES: 75   2 G PROTEIN   35 MG CHOLESTEROL
    12 G CARBOHYDRATES

Strawberry Angel Trifle

❦

1 large (8 servings) package sugar-free strawberry gelatin

1 angel food cake, about 8 inches in diameter

*20-ounce package frozen strawberries (no sugar added),
partially thawed*

*1 large (8 servings) package sugar-free vanilla pudding mix
(not instant)*

2¾ cups low-fat (2 percent) milk

1 cup "lite" frozen whipped topping, thawed

½ cup chopped nuts, such as walnuts

1. Prepare gelatin as directed on package. Refrigerate until syrupy.
2. Slice cake into thin pieces and line bottom of a 9-by-13-inch pan. Layer strawberries over cake, then top with syrupy gelatin mixture. Refrigerate until firm.
3. Prepare pudding per package directions, using 2¾ cups milk. Cool. Spread pudding on top of gelatin and strawberry layer. Refrigerate about 4 hours. Top with whipped topping and nuts.

YIELD: 12 SERVINGS
SERVING SIZE: ¹⁄₁₂ TRIFLE
CALORIES: 185
EXCHANGES: 1 FRUIT; 1 STARCH/BREAD; ¼ FAT

Strawberry Pineapple Parfait

❦

1 small (4 servings) package sugar-free strawberry gelatin
1 cup boiling water
1 cup sugar-free vanilla frozen yogurt or ice milk
½ cup crushed pineapple, in its own juice, drained
¾ cup frozen strawberries, no sugar added, thawed

Prepare gelatin, using 1 cup boiling water. Add frozen yogurt and fruits. Stir gently until well mixed. Refrigerate until ready to serve, at least 2 hours. Do not freeze.

YIELD: 2 CUPS;
4 SERVINGS
SERVING SIZE: ½ CUP
CALORIES: 75
EXCHANGES: 1 FRUIT;
½ FAT

1.5 G FAT
0.7 G FIBER
3.1 G PROTEIN
13.2 G CARBOHYDRATES

29 MG SODIUM
204 MG POTASSIUM
5 MG CHOLESTEROL

SAUCES, JAMS, AND SEASONINGS

Herb Seasoning for Fish

🌿

4 teaspoons "lite" margarine, melted

1 tablespoon Worcestershire sauce

1 tablespoon finely chopped onion

1 teaspoon parsley flakes

¼ teaspoon basil, dried

¼ teaspoon celery powder

½ teaspoon salt

dash ground pepper

Combine all ingredients. Spread over fish fillets before cooking. (*Note:* Other herbs of your choice may be combined, according to your taste.)

YIELD: 4 TABLESPOONS
SERVING SIZE: 1 TABLESPOON
CALORIES: A FREE FOOD

Saltless "Salt"

❦

1 teaspoon garlic powder

1 teaspoon onion powder

1 teaspoon paprika

1 teaspoon white pepper

1 teaspoon dry mustard

½ teaspoon thyme

½ teaspoon ground celery powder or celery seed

Mix all ingredients well, and store in a tightly covered container in a cool, dry place.

Herb Mixture

1 tablespoon garlic powder
1 teaspoon onion powder
1 teaspoon basil, dry
1 teaspoon chopped parsley, dry
1 teaspoon sage, dry
1 teaspoon savory, dry
1 teaspoon thyme, dry
1 teaspoon mace
1 teaspoon black pepper
½ teaspoon red pepper, dry

Mix all ingredients well, and store in a tightly covered container in a cool, dry place.

Whipped Topping

½ cup nonfat dry milk powder

½ cup ice water

1 teaspoon sugar substitute

1 teaspoon sugar

½ teaspoon vanilla extract

Chill small bowl and electric mixer beaters. Combine powdered milk with ice water in bowl. Beat until stiff. Add the sugar substitute, sugar, and vanilla. Serve immediately.

YIELD: 2 CUPS; 16 SERVINGS
SERVING SIZE: 2 TABLESPOONS
CALORIES: 10
EXCHANGES: FREE FOOD

Whipped Cream

¾ cup nonfat milk

1 cup nonfat cottage cheese

1 tablespoon vanilla extract

Combine ingredients in a blender at medium-high speed until frothy.

Cranberry Relish

✿

4 cups fresh or frozen cranberries
1 cup unsweetened orange juice
8 packets sugar substitute

In a saucepan, cook the cranberries with the orange juice until mixture thickens. Add the sugar substitute. Cover and refrigerate until ready to serve.

YIELD: 4½ CUPS
SERVING SIZE: ½ CUP
CALORIES: 35
EXCHANGES: 1 FRUIT

Grape Jelly

✿

1 envelope unflavored gelatin
¾ cup cold water
6-ounce can frozen unsweetened grape juice concentrate,
undiluted, thawed

Sprinkle gelatin in cold water, stirring until softened, about 1 minute. Add grape juice concentrate. Cook and stir until mixture boils. Store in a covered jar in the refrigerator.

YIELD: 1½ CUPS
CALORIES: 17.5 PER TABLESPOON
0.3 G PROTEIN
4.2 G CARBOHYDRATES

Beef Gravy

2 low-sodium beef bouillon cubes
1 cup boiling water
1 tablespoon minced onion
1 tablespoon cornstarch
¼ cup cold water
⅛ teaspoon salt
⅛ teaspoon pepper

In a small saucepan, combine bouillon cubes, boiling water, and minced onion. Simmer gently for 3 minutes. Combine cornstarch and cold water, stirring until well blended. Add to boiling bouillon, stirring constantly. Cook and stir over medium heat until smooth. Stir in salt and pepper.

YIELD: 1 CUP
SERVING SIZE: ¼ CUP
CALORIES: 11
EXCHANGES: UP TO ¼ CUP IS A FREE FOOD

Chicken Gravy

2 chicken bouillon cubes (low-sodium if desired)

1 cup boiling water

1 teaspoon minced onion

1 tablespoon cornstarch

¼ cup cold water

⅛ teaspoon salt

⅛ teaspoon pepper

In a small saucepan, combine bouillon cubes, boiling water, and onion. Simmer gently for 3 minutes, stirring occasionally. Combine cornstarch and cold water, stirring until well blended. Add to boiling bouillon, stirring constantly. Cook and stir over medium heat until thick and smooth. Stir in salt and pepper.

YIELD: 1 CUP; 4 SERVINGS
SERVING SIZE: ¼ CUP
CALORIES: 11
EXCHANGES: UP TO ¼ CUP IS A FREE FOOD

Spicy Party Dip

❧

1½ cups all-natural grape jelly
2 tablespoons cinnamon candies
2 tablespoons lemon juice
2 tablespoons catsup

Combine all ingredients in a saucepan and simmer until candies are melted. Serve hot in a bowl for dipping, with tiny meatballs, beef, or sausages; or pour over hot dogs or bratwurst in buns.

YIELD: 1¾ CUPS
SERVING SIZE: 1 TEASPOON
CALORIES: FREE FOOD
EXCHANGES: UP TO 1 TEASPOON IS A FREE FOOD

Spicy Dip

❦

8 ounces nonfat sour cream substitute

½ green pepper, chopped

1 bunch green onions, chopped, or 1 regular onion, chopped

½ jalapeño pepper, seeded, chopped

½ cup mild salsa

½ cup grated low-fat cheddar cheese

1 tomato, chopped

Layer ingredients in a serving dish, in order given, and serve with fat-free potato chips or other chips.

YIELD: 12 SERVINGS OR 3½ CUPS   LESS THAN ½ G FAT
SERVING SIZE: SCANT ⅓ CUP
CALORIES: 15 (PLUS CALORIES OF CHIPS)

Peach Jam

❦

48 ounces canned sliced peaches, in their own juice, drained;
reserve juice

1 envelope unflavored gelatin

½ cup sugar, or ¼ cup sugar and sugar substitute
equivalent to ¼ cup of sugar

Puree drained peaches in a blender. Measure puree and add enough juice to make 3 cups. Set aside. Measure another ¼ cup of juice into a saucepan. Sprinkle gelatin on juice. When gelatin is softened, add sugar and sugar substitute and heat to boiling, stirring constantly, until gelatin is completely dissolved. Combine with peach puree. Store in covered jar in refrigerator or freezer.

YIELD: 4 CUPS   0.3 G PROTEIN
CALORIES: 17 PER TABLESPOON   4.0 G CARBOHYDRATES

Fresh Raspberry Jam

1 tablespoon unflavored gelatin
2 tablespoons cold water
3 pints fresh raspberries or other fresh berries, crushed
¼ cup sugar
sugar substitute equivalent to ¾ cup sugar
1½ teaspoons lemon juice
½ cup liquid pectin

Soften the gelatin in the cold water. Combine berries with sugar, sugar substitute, and lemon juice in a saucepan. Heat to boiling and cook for 1 minute, stirring constantly. Stir in pectin and gelatin. Boil for 3 minutes, stirring constantly. Pour into jelly glasses. Cover and store in the refrigerator.

YIELD: 2 CUPS   0.2 G FAT
CALORIES: 43 PER TABLESPOON   0.6 G PROTEIN
       10.7 G CARBOHYDRATES

Mock Sour Cream

❦

2 tablespoons skim or low-fat (2 percent) milk
1 tablespoon lemon juice
1 cup low-fat sour cream or cottage cheese

Put all ingredients into a blender and mix until smooth and creamy. This may be added to hot dishes just before serving, or it may be served cold with herbs as a salad dressing.

YIELD: 8 SERVINGS
SERVING SIZE: ¼ CUP
CALORIES: 10
EXCHANGES: ¼ CUP = 1 FAT

Bert's Barbecue Sauce

❧

This is excellent with beef, pork, and chicken.

¼ cup vinegar

½ cup water

1 tablespoon sugar

1 packet sugar substitute

1 tablespoon prepared mustard

1 teaspoon salt

½ teaspoon black pepper

¼ teaspoon cayenne pepper

1 thick slice of lemon, or 2 tablespoons lemon juice

½ onion, thinly sliced

¼ cup margarine

½ cup catsup

2 tablespoons Worcestershire sauce

1½ teaspoons liquid smoke

Mix vinegar, water, sugar, sugar substitute, mustard, salt, pepper, cayenne pepper, lemon, onion, and margarine in a saucepan. Simmer uncovered for 20 minutes. Add the catsup, Worcestershire sauce, and liquid smoke and bring to a boil for 2 minutes. Store in the refrigerator, covered.

YIELD: 1¾ CUPS
SERVING SIZE: ⅛ (2 TABLESPOONS)
CALORIES: 30

Microwave Salsa

28-ounce can whole tomatoes; drained; reserve juice
4-ounce can chopped green chilies
1 cup chopped onion
2 tablespoons cooking oil
2 teaspoons cumin
½ teaspoon crushed red chili flakes

Pour reserved tomato juice into a 2-quart casserole. Chop tomatoes and add to juice. Stir in remaining ingredients. Microwave at high for 8 to 10 minutes or until flavors are well blended. Serve as a dip with nacho chips or spoon over tacos, enchiladas, or burritos.

YIELD: 4 CUPS
SERVING SIZE: ¼ CUP
CALORIES: 40
EXCHANGES: 2 VEGETABLE

Orange and Lemon Sauce

❦

This is excellent over angel food cake, frozen yogurt, or other desserts.

1 cup unsweetened orange juice
¼ cup lemon juice
⅔ cup water
2 tablespoons cornstarch
3 tablespoons sugar
sugar substitute equivalent to ½ cup sugar

In a saucepan, combine all ingredients except sugar and sugar substitute. Cook over medium heat, stirring constantly. Bring to a boil and continue cooking for 2 minutes longer. Remove from heat and cool slightly. Add sugars and stir gently.

YIELD: 2 CUPS
SERVING SIZE: ¼ CUP (4 TABLESPOONS)
CALORIES: 60
EXCHANGES: 4 TABLESPOONS = 1 FRUIT

Pink Applesauce

3 cups sliced apples, such as Ida red or Cortland
12 cinnamon-flavored red candies

Place apples in a microwavable dish and cook at medium setting for 8 minutes. Stir in candies and microwave 2 minutes longer, or until candies are dissolved.

YIELD: 6 SERVINGS
SERVING SIZE: ½ CUP
CALORIES: 60
EXCHANGES: 1 FRUIT; ¼ FAT

Quick Strawberry Sauce

10-ounce package frozen, unsweetened strawberries, thawed,crushed, and drained; reserve juice
1 tablespoon cornstarch

Blend reserved juice and cornstarch in a small saucepan. Heat to boiling, stirring constantly. Boil for 1 minute. Remove from heat. Stir in strawberries and cool completely. Spoon over frozen yogurt or ice milk. Store tightly covered in refrigerator for up to 1 week.

YIELD: 1 CUP
SERVING SIZE: 1 TABLESPOON
CALORIES: 10.5
EXCHANGES: ½ FRUIT
2.7 G CARBOHYDRATES

GLOSSARY

Bake:	Cook in oven.
Baste:	Moisten food with liquid during cooking to add flavor.
Beat:	Stir briskly, around and around vertically.
Blend:	Mix two or more ingredients together.
Broil:	Cook by direct heat from above, as in a broiler.
Brown:	Brown meat in a frying pan, until pinkness is gone.
Chop:	Cut into small pieces with a chopper or knife.
Cream:	To beat into a creamy, light, and fluffy consistency: for example, shortening and eggs.
Dash:	Less than ⅛ teaspoon of any ingredient.
Dice:	Cut into very small pieces.
Dust:	Sprinkle pan lightly with flour.
Dutch oven:	Large, heavy cooking kettle with tight-fitting cover.
Fold:	Combine ingredients together gently, bringing spoon through a mixture, across bottom and up sides of bowl. Broader and slower than beating.
Fry:	Cook in hot oil or shortening.

Knead:	Use hands to work dough.
Marinate:	Let ingredients stand in a liquid to enhance flavors.
Mash:	To stir or use masher to make a soft mass; example: to mash potatoes.
Mince:	Chop very fine. Diced is finer than chopped, minced is finer than diced.
Puree:	Food processed in a blender or pressed through a sieve to form a smooth consistency.
Sauté:	In a frying pan, spray a small amount of cooking spray. Cut vegetables into thin slices, add ½ cup liquid and flavorings and cook until done. There should be very little liquid remaining when they are done.
Shred:	Tear or cut into small pieces.
Simmer:	Cook in liquid over low heat without boiling.
Stir-fry:	Cut meat into bite-size pieces, slice vegetables very thin. In a frying pan or wok, add a small amount of cooking oil, add meat and vegetables. Cover with ½ cup water. This cooks very quickly.
Tester or Cake tester:	A toothpick or knife, inserted in the middle of breads or cakes to test doneness.
Toss:	Mix lightly.
Whip:	Beat rapidly to increase volume, as egg whites.
Wire whisk:	Kitchen utensil used to mix with a back-and-forth, round-and-round motion.

Suggestions

- Buy a good can opener.
- Buy an egg separator—the yolk stays in the top and the white goes into a bottom unit.
- Buy a pastry brush.
- Buy a pizza cutter.
- Buy a pair of tongs.

Appendix A

NUTRITIONAL CONTENTS

BASIC MEAL COMPOSITION

Protein food

Starch food

Fruit

Fiber (vegetable, whole grain)

Small amount of fat

For good nutrition choose a variety of foods:

Protein Foods

(lean cuts of beef, pork, lamb, skinned poultry, low-fat cheeses, peanut butter, select grades of red meats)

- Have 1 to 2 ounces at breakfast and a 3-ounce portion at lunch and dinner.
- Limit red meats to one meal a day and keep egg yolks to 2 to 3 per week if your cholesterol is high.

Starchy Vegetables and Breads/Cereals

(whole-grain breads, rolls, rice, pastas, potatoes, squash, peas, corn, crackers, oats, legumes [dried beans and peas])

- Have 4 or more servings per day.
- Eat the same number of servings at each meal.

Fruits

(fresh, frozen, or canned in fruit juice or water)

- Have 2 to 4 servings per day with 1 serving of a fruit high in vitamin C (citrus, melons, berries).
- Leave skins and seeds on fruits—they add fiber and help control blood sugar.
- Allow only small (2 tablespoons) amount of juice in a serving of juice-packed canned fruit.
- Avoid drinking juices because they make blood sugar skyrocket.
- Always include fruit as a part of a meal. Never eat fruit alone.
- Watch the portion size. Lots of fruit means a high blood sugar.

Vegetables

(fresh, frozen, or canned)

- Have 2 to 4 servings per day.
- Choose fresh or frozen more often to increase fiber in your diet.
- Cook in small amounts of water until just tender.
- Choose more deep green and yellow vegetables and cruciferous vegetables (cabbage family) for vitamin A and beta carotene.

Fats

(soft tub margarine, salad dressings, oils, low-fat cream cheese)

- Limit fats to 2 to 5 teaspoons a day.
- Avoid solid fats, especially meat fats and high-fat dairy foods.
- Use more liquid oils and soft margarine in cooking and as a spread.

- Avoid fried foods.
- Look for polyunsaturated/saturated fat ratio on package labels. A 2-to-1 ratio is recommended.

Milk

- 2 cups per day for adults of skim or 2 percent low-fat milk.
- For children and adolescents, 3 to 4 cups per day of 2 percent low-fat milk.
- Drink milk with meals. Taken as a snack, milk will make blood sugar climb.

Salt

- Try cutting down on the amount in cooking and at the table.
- Limit salty foods.

Alcohol

Follow physician's advice. Alcohol causes blood sugar to drop quickly, so consume cocktails, wine, beer, and other spirits with meals only. Avoid all alcohol if your doctor advises it.

Free Foods

Foods that you can consume in unlimited amounts include coffee and tea (regular and decaffeinated), diet soda pop, broth or bouillon, dill pickles, sugarless gum, diet jellies and syrups, diet gelatin and pudding, sugar-free popsicles, vinegar, lemon juice, herbs, and spices.

Low-Sugar Treats

- Low-sugar cookies, such as vanilla wafers, Lorna Doones™, shortbread, graham crackers, gingersnaps, and animal crackers

- Cake or yeast-raised doughnuts (no sugar or glaze)
- Ice cream or frozen yogurt (chocolate, vanilla, and strawberry)—limit to twice a week
- Pies with filling artificially sweetened or with no sugar added
- Sugarless candies (in moderation)
- Fruit spreads (such as Simply Fruit™)

Consume in moderate amounts as part of a meal or snack.

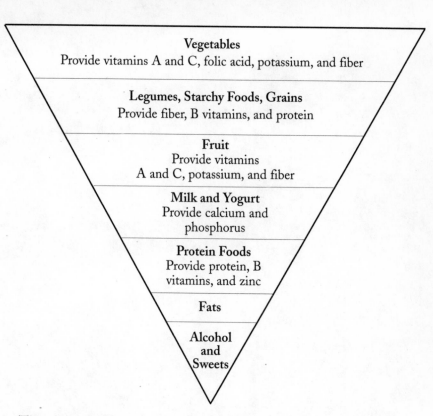

Vegetables
Provide vitamins A and C, folic acid, potassium, and fiber

Legumes, Starchy Foods, Grains
Provide fiber, B vitamins, and protein

Fruit
Provide vitamins
A and C, potassium, and fiber

Milk and Yogurt
Provide calcium and
phosphorus

Protein Foods
Provide protein, B
vitamins, and zinc

Fats

**Alcohol
and
Sweets**

This diagram illustrates the food groups and the key nutrients in each group. You can also use the diagram to determine which foods you need to include the most of in your daily diet. Vegetables are on top and should lead the way in food choices. Fats, alcohol, and sweets are on the bottom and provide lots of calories for the few nutrients they contain. In fact, alcohol is truly the "empty" calorie because it robs the body of nutrients and offers none in return.

Source: American Diabetes Association

Appendix B

FOOD LISTS

MILK LIST

(nonfat [skim] and low-fat milk)

One nonfat choice provides:

0 g fat

12 g carbohydrates

8 g protein

80 calories

Nonfat Choices

Nonfat (skim) milk

Powdered, nonfat milk (before adding liquid)

Sugar-free hot cocoa mix plus 6 ounces water

One low-fat choice provides:

3 g fat

12 g carbohydrates

8 g protein

107 calories

Low-Fat Choices

Low-fat milk (1%)

Yogurt, plain, unflavored, made from skim milk

FAT LIST

(butter, margarine, cream, mayonnaise, nuts, salad dressings, vegetable oils, and other fatty foods)

One choice provides:

5 g fat

45 calories

Best for Your Heart and Blood Vessels

Margarine: soft, tub, or stick

Mayonnaise: reduced-calorie

Nuts: almonds, peanuts, walnuts

Oils: corn, cottonseed, safflower, soy, sunflower, olive, peanut

Olives: green or black

Salad dressings: French, Italian, mayonnaise-type

Not as Good for Your Heart and Blood Vessels

Bacon

Butter

Coffee whitener, liquid

Cool Whip™

Cream: half-and-half, sour cream

Cream cheese: whipped or "lite"

MEAT LIST

(meat, fish, poultry, eggs, cheese, and meat substitutes)

One low-fat choice provides:

3 g fat

7 g protein

55 calories

Low-Fat Choices

Cheese: cottage, pot, 1% fat, Lite-Line™, Nuform™, Weight Watchers™

Canned: water-packed salmon or tuna; water-packed clams, oysters, scallops, shrimp; sardines, drained

Fresh or frozen: fish and seafood

Luncheon meat: 95% fat-free

Poultry: chicken, turkey, or Cornish hen, without skin

One medium-fat choice provides:

5 g fat

7 g protein

75 calories

Medium-Fat Choices

Cheese: skim or part-skim milk cheese; Parmesan, Romano

Beef: chipped, chuck, flank steak, hamburger with 15% fat, rib eye, rump sirloin, tender-loin top, and bottom round

Lamb

Pork, except for deviled ham, ground pork, and spareribs

Veal

Eggs

Egg substitutes

One high-fat choice provides:

8 g fat

7 g protein

100 calories

High-Fat Choices

These protein foods are high in fat. Do not use them often.

Regular cheese: blue, Brie, cheddar, Colby feta, Monterey Jack, Muenster, provolone, Swiss, pasteurized process

Fried fish

Beef: brisket, club and rib steaks, corned beef, regular hamburger with 20% fat, rib roast, short ribs

Frankfurters

Luncheon meats: Bologna, bratwurst, braunschweiger, knockwurst, liverwurst, pastrami,

Organ meats: liver, heart, kidney

Polish sausage, salami

Pork: deviled ham, ground pork, spareribs, sausage (patty or link)

STARCH/BREAD LIST

(bread, crackers, cereal, pasta, starchy vegetables, and other starchy food items)

One choice provides:
trace of fat
15 g carbohydrates
3 g protein
80 calories

Breads

(in general, one choice equals 1 ounce of bread)

Bagel
English muffin
Reduced-calorie: (1 slice equals 40 calories)
Rolls: dinner, plain; hamburger
Syrian pita pocket, 6-inch diameter
White, whole-wheat, or rye

Cereals

(one choice equals ½ cup)

Cooked cereals
Bran: All Bran™*, 40%
Bran Flakes™*, Bran Chex™
Cheerios™
Cornflakes™
Nutrigrain™, wheat

Puffed rice or wheat
Rice Krispies™
Shredded Wheat™ biscuit*
   spoon-size
Special K™
Sunflakes™

Cereals high in fiber

Starchy Vegetables

Corn	Potato, white, mashed or baked
Lima beans	Sweet potato, mashed or baked
Peas, green, canned or frozen	Winter squash: acorn or butternut

Pasta (cooked)

Macaroni, noodles, spaghetti

Dried Beans, Peas, and Lentils

Baked beans, canned, no pork (vegetarian style)
Beans, peas, lentils (dried and cooked)

Prepared Foods

Biscuit, 2-inch diameter (1 ounce)
Cornbread, 2-by-2-by-1 inches
Croissant, 4-by-4-by-1¾ inches
Muffin, bran or corn, 2-inch diameter (1½ ounces)
Pancake, 4-inch diameter
Waffle, 4-inch diameter

Others

Bread crumbs
Potato or macaroni salad
Rice, cooked

Occasional Choices

These foods are high in fat. Do not use more than two times a week.

French fries, 2- to 3½-inch length   Popcorn, popped in oil

Ice cream   Potato or corn chips

Popcorn, microwave   Stuffing mix, cooked

Crackers (equal to one bread choice)

Gingersnaps

Graham crackers

2½-inch squares

Matzoh™

Melba™ toast rectangles

Pretzel sticks

Rice cakes

Rye Krisp™, three triple crackers

Saltine™ crackers

Stella D'Oro Egg Biscuit™

Uneedas™

Wasa Lite™ or Golden Rye
   Crisp Bread™

Crackers (equal to one bread plus one fat choice)

These crackers are high in fat. Count them as one bread choice plus one fat choice.

Cheez-its™

Club™ or Townhouse™ crackers

Peanut Butter Sandwich Crackers™

Pepperidge Farm Goldfish™

Ritz™

Stella D'Oro Breakfast Treats™

Stella D'Oro Sesame
   Breadsticks™

Triscuits™

Vanilla Wafers™

Wasa Sesame™ or
   Breakfast Crisp Bread™

Wheat Thins™

VEGETABLE LIST

(fresh, frozen, and canned vegetables)

One choice provides:

5 g carbohydrates

2 g protein

28 calories

Vegetables

Asparagus	Mushrooms, fresh
Beets	Spinach, cooked
Broccoli	Squash, summer or zucchini
Carrots	Tomato, ripe
Cauliflower	Tomato sauce, canned
Green beans	Vegetables, mixed

Low-Calorie Vegetables

These vegetables are low in calories. You may have as much as you want if you eat them raw.

Alfalfa sprouts	Lettuce
Chicory	Parsley
Chinese cabbage	Pickles, unsweetened
Cucumber	Pimento
Endive	Spinach
Escarole	Watercress

FRUIT LIST

(fresh fruit, pure fruit juices, and canned, dried, cooked, or frozen fruit without extra sugar)

One choice provides:
15 g carbohydrates
60 calories

Fruits

Apple, 2-inch diameter

Banana, 9-inch length

Blueberries

Cantaloupe, 5-inch diameter, sectioned, cubed

Grapefruit, 4-inch diameter

Grapes

Nectarine, 2½-inch diameter

Orange, 3-inch diameter

Peach, 2½-inch diameter, fresh, canned*

Pear, fresh, canned*

Pineapple, canned*

Prunes, dried, medium

Raisins

Strawberries

Tangerine, 2½-inch diameter

Watermelon, diced

Do not use the liquid from canned fruit.

FOODS USING MORE THAN ONE FOOD GROUP

Canned Soup

Cream soup made with water

Minestrone, ready-to-serve

Rice or noodle with broth prepared with water

Tomato, made with water

Other Foods

Beef stew, homemade

Chili with meat and beans, homemade

Plain cheese pizza

Pudding, sugar-free, made with skim or 1% low-fat milk

Ravioli, canned

FREE FOOD GROUP

These foods are low in calories. You may have as much as you want unless otherwise noted.

Bouillon cubes	Mustard, prepared
Calorie-free soft drinks	Pickles, unsweetened
Catsup (1 tablespoon daily)	Soy sauce
Coffee	Spices
Herbs	Tea
Horseradish	Vinegar

FOODS LIKELY TO CAUSE PROBLEMS

These foods are high in sugar and may cause high blood sugar. Do not use them unless your dietitian or doctor says you can.

Alcohol*: sweet wines, liqueurs, cordials

Candy

Carbonated beverages containing sugar (including "natural" sodas)

Chewing gum (regular)

Dates, figs, and other dried fruits

Desserts containing sugar: cakes; cookies with filling or frosting; ice cream, including sodas and sundaes; ice milk; gelatin desserts, sweetened; pies; puddings; sherbet

Fructose

Fruited yogurt

Honey

Jam and jelly (nondietetic)

Marmalade

Pastries

Preserves

Sugar

Sugar-coated cereals

Sugar-sweetened fruit drinks (Kool-Aid™, Hi-C™, etc.)

Sweetened condensed milk

Syrups (maple, molasses, etc.)

*Avoid all alcohol unless your doctor or dietitian advises otherwise.
Source: Presbyterian Diabetes Center of Albuquerque

RECIPE MODIFICATIONS

Don't throw out your favorite recipe! Below is a list of possible low-fat, sodium and sugar substitutions that can be used to make your recipes healthier. Try adapting some of your old favorites using recipe modifications.

Most important: Be creative and positive and keep repeating the recipe until you "get it right."

INGREDIENTS	POSSIBLE SUBSTITUTIONS
Butter, margarine, or cooking oil	The availability of nonstick frying pans makes nonfat cooking possible. Nonstick vegetable sprays work well to prevent sticking. Replace fat with equal amounts of defatted stocks (beef, chicken, or vegetable), wine, juice, water, or other liquids. Fats can be left out of soups, stews, and casseroles. To remove any fat, chill in refrigerator for several hours and remove congealed fat. Each tablespoon of oil eliminated reduces calories by 100.
Cakes, cookies, pastries	Homemade bran muffins or quick bread. Make your own sweet treats by using whole-grain flours, such as oatmeal, and reduce fat.

Chocolate	Carob powder is low in fat and contains no caffeine. Unsweetened, it is suitable in many recipes. Three to 4 tablespoons carob powder worked into 1 tablespoon skim milk and 1 tablespoon oil is equal to 1 ounce chocolate. When converting a recipe from chocolate to carob, reduce the amount of sweetener to compensate for carob's natural sweetness. Reduce the oven temperature 25° to avoid over-browning. Avoid carob chips which contain palm oil, and carob candy bars, which are full of added sugar and fat.
Egg (1 whole)	2 egg whites, or ¼ cup egg substitute.
1 egg yolk	1 egg white
Ground beef	Use lower-fat ground round, veal, venison, or turkey. Cut down on the amount of meat and increase vegetables. Precooked legumes such as kidney beans also work well in casseroles or stews.
Light or heavy cream	Replace all or part of the cream with evaporated skim milk.
Nondairy creamer	Evaporated skim milk
Nuts	Raisins
Salad dressing	Standard salad dressing recipes call for a 3–1 ratio of oil to vinegar. This can be easily reduced to 2-1 or 1-1. The ratio will depend on the kind of vinegar used and the other ingredients. Balsamic

vinegar, a mild Italian vinegar, or rice vinegar need very little oil to produce a tasty dressing.

Salt

Experiment with the use of more herbs and spices to reduce or eliminate salt. Wine, sherry, and low-sodium bouillon add flavor to foods. Prepared mustard and horseradish are excellent flavor additions; use sparingly because they contain some sodium.

Sour cream or mayonnaise (1 cup)

1 cup plain yogurt; or 1 cup "Mock Sour Cream" (see recipe on page 200). Use as a substitute in dips, dressings, desserts, sauces, baking, soups, or marinades.

Tofu

A vegetable cheese made from soy milk, which contains no cholesterol. A 3.5-ounce serving of tofu has 72 calories. Tofu has a bland taste, but absorbs the flavor of foods with which it is combined. Cubed it is a good substitute for chicken or meat; blended, it is a good substitute for cheese.

Wheat flour (1 cup)

¾ cup buckwheat; or ¾ cup coarse cornmeal; or 1 scant cup fine cornmeal; or ¾ cup rye flour; or 1⅓ cups oatmeal

White flour (1 cup all-purpose)

1 cup whole-wheat flour minus 2 tablespoons; or ½ cup white and ½ cup whole-wheat flour; or ¾ cup white flour and ¼ cup bran

White sauce	Eliminate the fat and blend unbleached flour or cornstarch with nonfat milk as usual; season to taste. You will reduce calories if you use cornstarch or arrowroot in place of flour; you'll require only about half as much.
Whole milk	Nonfat milk (add extra nonfat dry milk powder to liquid milk for a thicker consistency; you save 72 calories per cup by using skim milk.

BAKED GOODS

There's no need to give up your favorite baked goods to eat leaner. Here's how to reduce the fat in your recipes by one-third to one-half without losing the great taste:

For a Tasty Dessert	Use This Much Fat
Cakes and soft-drop cookies	No more than 2 tablespoons of fat per cup of flour
Muffins, quick breads, biscuits	No more than 1 to 2 tablespoons of fat per cup of flour
Pie crust	½ cup margarine for 2 cups flour

DESSERT AND BEVERAGE CHOICES

Instead Of	Choose
Apple or cherry pie	Custard or pumpkin pie
Candy bar	Ice cream or ice milk

Chocolate cake or torte	Angel food or pound cake
Cranberry sauce	Cranberries + sugar substitute
Fruit canned in sugar syrup	Fruit canned in water or syrup juice
Fruit-flavored yogurt	Plain yogurt + sugar substitute
Fruit gelatin	Sugar-free gelatin
Pancake syrup	Applesauce (unsweetened)
Sugar in coffee or tea	Sugar substitute in coffee or tea
Sweetened soft drinks	Diet soft drinks

Source: Memorial Medical Center of West Michigan

LOW-FAT SUBSTITUTES

Substitute the following low-fat foods for high-fat ones

High-Fat Foods	Low-Fat Foods
Avocado	Cucumber; zucchini; lettuce
Bacon	Chicken (or Canadian bacon)
Bologna, frankfurter, sausage	Chicken or turkey; lean, thinly sliced beef
Breakfast sausage	Toast with cottage cheese
Chocolate	Candy (if you must have it) that contains no chocolate; sweet wafers made with no fat
Cream	Skim milk
Cream pie	Unfrosted cake, made with less fat than the recipe calls for
Creamy or high-fat cheese	Low-fat cheese; cottage cheese
Fast-food meal on a long car trip	Pack a homemade meal of lean broiled chicken, fruits, and raw vegetables
Fatty pork (spareribs, ground pork)	Well-trimmed lean pork, (leg, ham)

Fried egg	Poached or baked egg
Ground beef	Extra-lean or lean beef with all fat trimmed
Hot chocolate or chocolate milk (made with whole milk)	Hot chocolate or chocolate milk made with skim or low-fat milk; strawberry or raspberry syrup mixed into skim or low-fat milk; lemonade; fruit juice; skim milk blended with raw fruit such as bananas or strawberries
Hot dogs and hamburgers at a cookout	Chicken; skewered shrimp; broiled fish
Hot fudge sundae	Frozen yogurt or ice milk with sliced or crushed fruit
Ice cream	Ice milk; frozen low-fat yogurt
Liver	Lean meat; chicken; fish; veal; low-fat cheese
Nuts	Fruit or vegetable snack
Oil or mayonnaise dressing on cold pasta salad	Tomato sauce; yogurt laced with herbs
Peanut butter and jelly sandwich	Turkey breast; chicken; water-packed tuna; crabmeat or shrimp salad; low-fat cheese
Potato chips	Raw vegetables; whole-grain crackers; pretzels

Regular salad dressing	Reduced-calorie salad dressing; vinegar; lemon juice
Sardines	Shrimp; crabmeat; lobster
Sour cream	Low-fat yogurt; imitation sour cream
Whipped cream	Whipped evaporated skim milk (the bowl and beaters must be thoroughly chilled)
Whole milk	Skim milk; buttermilk; nonfat powdered milk

Source: Memorial Medical Center of West Michigan

Appendix E

SUGAR SUBSTITUTIONS AND ARTIFICIAL SWEETENER EQUIVALENCIES

SUGAR SUBSTITUTES

In the United States, the three major sugar substitutes are: aspartame (Equal™, NutraSweet™, NutraSweet Spoonful™); saccharin (Sweet 'N Low™, Sugar Twin™, Sprinkle Sweet™); and acesulfame K (Sweet One™).

Aspartame must be added after cooking. I prefer acesulfame K for baking and cooking.

Amount of Artificial Sweeteners to Substitute for Sugar

Sugar	Acesulfame K	Aspartame	Saccharin
2 teaspoons	1 packet	1 packet	1 packet
1 tablespoon	1¼ packets	1½ packets	1⅓ packets
¼ cup	3 packets	6 packets	3 packets
⅓ cup	4 packets	8 packets	4 packets
1 cup	12 packets	24 packets	12 packets

SUGAR WORD LIST

All the below are sugars:

Brown sugar	Maltodextrin
Corn syrup	Maltose
Corn syrup solids	Maple syrup
Corn sweetners	Molasses
Crystalline fructose	Natural carbohydrates
Dextrose	Raw sugar
Fruit sugar	Sorghum
High fructose corn syrup	Sucrose
Honey	Turbinado

Source: Presbyterian Diabetes Center of Albuquerque

EQUIVALENCIES FOR ARTIFICIAL SWEETENERS

Sweetener	Amount	Sugar Equivalent
Sprinkle Sweet™	1 teaspoon	1 teaspoon
Sugar Twin™	1 teaspoon	1 teaspoon
Sugar Twin™, *Brown*	1 teaspoon	1 teaspoon
Sweet 'N Low™	¹⁄₁₀ teaspoon	1 teaspoon
	⅓ teaspoon	1 tablespoon
	1 teaspoon	⅙ cup
	½ teaspoon	¼ cup
	1 tablespoon	½ cup
	2 tablespoons	1 cup

Sweetener	Amount	Sugar Equivalent
Adolph's Sugar Substitute™	2 shakes of jar	1 rounded teaspoon
	¼ teaspoon	1 tablespoon
	1 teaspoon	¼ cup
	2½ teaspoons	⅔ cup
	1 tablespoon	¾ cup
	4 teaspoons	1 cup
Sucaryl™(liquid sweetener)	⅛ teaspoon	1 teaspoon
	⅜ teaspoon	1 tablespoon
	¾ teaspoon	2 tablespoons
	1½ teaspoons	¼ cup
	1 tablespoon	½ cup
	2 tablespoons	1 cup
Weight Watchers Sweet'ner™	⅛ teaspoon	1 teaspoon
Sweet 10™, Liquid (6 drops = ⅛ teaspoon)	⅛ teaspoon	1 teaspoon
	¼ teaspoon	1 tablespoon
	1 teaspoon	¼ cup
	1 tablespoon	¾ cup
	4 teaspoons	1 cup
Sweet 10™, Tablets	1 tablet	1 teaspoon
	3 tablets	1 tablespoon
	12 tablets	¼ cup
	36 tablets	¾ cup
	48 tablets	1 cup
Equal™, Granulated	1 packet	2 teaspoons
Equal™, Tablets	1 tablet	1 teaspoon

Prepared by Liz DeShelter, Columbus, Ohio. Reprinted with permission from Diabetes Care and Education Newsletter, published by the American Dietetic Association. Consult your nutritionist before using any sweetener.

Appendix F

THE "50/50" PLATE: HOW DOES FOOD AFFECT BLOOD GLUCOSE?

BALANCE FOODS FOR GLYCEMIC EFFECT

Foods that increase blood glucose

Foods that slow blood glucose

Starch
Fruit
Milk

Meat/
protein
Vegetables
Salad

1. Draw an imaginary line down the middle of your plate. On the left side you can have servings of foods that increase blood glucose. These include: fruit, starch, or milk. On the right side of the plate you can have servings of foods that slow blood glucose. These may include: meat/protein, vegetables, or salad (using low-fat dressing). For every serving on the left side of the plate you must have a serving on the right side for "balance."

2. You can have only one meat/protein serving. This should be a lean meat, poultry, or fish that is not fried. If you use cheese, select the low-fat cheeses. A meat serving should be no more than 3 to 4 ounces, or about the size of the palm of your hand.

3. Use the 50/50 plate to balance snacks. Having some protein with your starch will balance your snacks as well. Use some peanut butter or cheese on crackers to slow the effect of the starch.

Source: Presbyterian Diabetes Center of Albuquerque

Carbohydrates (sugars and starches raise blood glucose quickly)

Sugars are mainly made up of glucose; they are digested and absorbed very fast. Sugars are found in white sugar and fruit sugar. Milk also contains lactose, which is a fast-acting carbohydrate.

Starches like crackers, bread, potatoes, and rice are broken down into glucose and absorbed quickly. Starches are long chains of glucose units. They can be hundreds of units long. Because of this complex structure, they are broken down a little more slowly than sugars, although many people notice that starches eaten alone cause a quick blood glucose rise. About 50 percent of a meal can be carbohydrate foods. This is a good balance that will provide enough glucose for fuel without causing high blood glucose.

Protein (meats, cheese, peanut butter, and tofu)

Protein foods help to slow down the breakdown of starch and fruit sugar. If crackers (starch) are combined with cheese or meat (protein), the mixed snack (starch and protein) slows digestion. A slow breakdown of food means glucose levels do not go too high. Some protein can be converted into blood glucose three hours after eating and helps to stabilize blood glucose control.

Fiber (helps control blood sugar)

There are two types of fiber.

- *Soluble fiber* absorbs water and becomes a gel. It helps to lower cholesterol. Sources of soluble fiber include oat bran and beans.
- *Insoluble fiber* absorbs water and increases in volume but does

not form a gel. It helps regulate lower bowel function and pre-
vents constipation. Insoluble fiber is found in bran and whole
grains, vegetables, and whole fruit.

Both types of fiber help to control blood glucose because they
slow digestion. Adding high-fiber foods to meals will give better
blood glucose control.

Fats (help control blood glucose)

A small amount of fat (about 1 teaspoon) is recommended at
each meal. Fat adds a satisfied feeling to the meal as well as slow-
ing digestion. Fats do not cause blood glucose levels to rise in
most people, although people with Type II diabetes will want to
eat less fat to reduce insulin resistance and for weight control.
Notice the different types of fats content among the protein
sources. There are three types: saturated, polyunsaturated, and
monosaturated. All types of fats have the same amount of calories, but they affect blood cholesterol differently.

- *Saturated fats* (meat fat, butter, lard, shortening, coconut, and
  palm oils): solid at room temperature and raise blood cholesterol.
- *Polyunsaturated fats* (soybean, safflower, sunflower, and corn
  oils): liquid at room temperature and lower cholesterol.
- *Monounsaturated fats* (peanut oil, canola oil, and olive oil): liquid at room temperature and lower cholesterol.

It is best to use more liquid fat, such as oils and soft mar-
garines, rather than solid fats. It is also wise to select lean meats
and poultry and fish to reduce fat so that it makes up less than 30
percent of total calories.

FOODS RICH IN POTASSIUM

Foods rich in potassium are necessary to a healthy diet. Normal level is 4 mg per 100 ccs of blood. Potassium quantities must be in balance with sodium quantities. Marked alterations occur with many diseases and may cause disturbance in heart function. Potassium helps muscle contraction and nerve transmission and helps maintain blood pressure. A potassium deficiency can cause muscle weakness, nausea, and heart problems. Have your potassium level checked when you have your annual physical. Studies are being conducted on how much potassium is healthy, but they are still inconclusive.

	Average Portion	Potassium (mg)	Calories
Fruits			
Apricots	3 medium	500	55
Avocado	½	380	275
Banana	1 medium	630	130
Cantaloupe	½ melon	880	75
Dates	1 cup	1390	500
Grapefruit	1 cup	380	75
Orange	1 medium	360	95
Prunes	4 large	240	90
Raisins	1 cup	1150	425
Strawberries	1 cup	270	55
Watermelon	½ slice	380	95

	Average Portion	Potassium (mg)	Calories
Juices			
Grapefruit	8 oz.	370	130
Orange	8 oz.	440	105
Pineapple	8 oz.	340	120
Prune	8 oz.	620	170
Meat			
Beef (chuck)	3 oz.	290	310
Beef (round)	3 oz.	310	260
Hamburger	3 oz.	340	200
Rib roast	3 oz.	290	270
Turkey	4 oz.	350	300
Vegetables			
Artichoke	1 medium	210	30
Brussel sprouts	1 cup	300	35
Tomato	1 medium	340	30

Appendix H

FOODS HIGH IN SODIUM

If your diet is to be restricted in sodium (salt), the following foods should be avoided unless they are labeled "low-sodium." Low-sodium foods are available on most supermarket shelves. If salt or sodium is listed as one of the first three ingredients in a product, do not buy it, as it is high in salt.

Meats and Fish

Avoid smoked, cured, or canned meats and fish, unless labeled "dietetic-low sodium."

Anchovies	Corned beef	Luncheon meats
Bacon	Frankfurters	Salt pork
Canned salmon	Ham	Sardines
Canned tuna	Herring	Sausage
Chicken franks	Kosher meats	Scrapple

Vegetables

Baked beans	Tomato juice
Pickles	Vegetable juice cocktail
Sauerkraut	Vegetables pickled in brine

Snack Foods

Avoid any salted snack food.

Corn chips	Potato chips	Salted popcorn
Olives	Pretzels	Snack crackers
Party dips	Salted nuts	Soda crackers

Sauces, Soups, Seasonings

Barbecue sauce	Canned soups (unless low-sodium)
Chili sauce	Instant and dried soups
Steak sauce	Meat tenderizers
Worcestershire sauce	Monosodium glutamate (MSG)
Bouillon	Seasoned salt (garlic, onion, celery)

Miscellaneous

Cheese

Frozen dinners

Most salt substitutes contain a large amount of potassium instead of sodium, so check that on labels, too. Do not consume more than 1,000 mg of sodium per 1,000 calories of your diet.

Instead of salt, try one or two herbs at a time until you find a combination that you like. Try the "Saltless 'Salt'" and "Herb Mixture" recipes on pages 190 and 191.

Herbs are a "free food" in your diet. Herbs differ from spices, which are made from the dried bark, roots, berries, and buds of plants that grow in a tropical climate. Herbs are made from the leaves of plants, and the leaves are the only part used in seasoning food.

Source: Presbyterian Diabetes Center of Albuquerque

Appendix I

ADDING FIBER TO YOUR DIET

You need fiber in your food to make you healthy. Most men and women eat only half of the fiber they need.

Eating More Fiber May Reduce Your Risk For:

- Heart disease
- Adult diabetes
- Cancer of the colon
- Obesity

Not Eating Enough Fiber in Your Diet, You May:

- Get hungry between meals
- Gain weight from fats and sweets
- Have problems with constipation
- Suffer from hemorrhoids

Foods Containing Fiber Can:

- Lower cholesterol
- Lower blood sugar
- Fill you up, not out
- Improve your health

How Does Fiber Taste?

• Crispy	Apples
• Hot	Peppers
• Juicy	Oranges
• Crunchy	Popcorn
• Sweet	Melons
• Smooth	Pinto beans

Fiber provides all these various tastes with only half the calories of fats and alcohol.

Which Foods Contain Fiber?

- Beans
- Dried Peas
- Fruits
- Nuts and seeds (high in fat)
- Vegetables
- Whole-grain breads and cereals

How to Eat More Fiber at Home

- Eat fruits and vegetables unpeeled.
- Use whole-grain flours in baking.
- Combine fiber foods with meat.
- Buy whole-grain breads and cereals.

How to Eat More Fiber Away from Home

- Include a salad or vegetable with your meal.
- Choose baked potatoes, beans, or rice.
- Order pizza with vegetable toppings.
- Enjoy popcorn for snacks.
- Add fiber-rich, low-fat toppings to salads or baked potatoes.

Remember

- Eat more fiber.
- Increase exercise.
- Choose lower-fat foods.
- Use less salt and sugar.
- Use alcohol in moderation.
- Be tobacco-free.
- Drink lots of water.

A healthy lifestyle is within your reach!

Source: Memorial Medical Center of West Michigan

Appendix J

HOW TO LOWER
YOUR CHOLESTEROL

How You Can Lower Your Cholesterol Risk

- Don't smoke. Smoking decreases HDL or "good cholesterol" levels in the bloodstream.
- Obtain or maintain a desirable weight.
- Exercise regularly. HDL levels can be raised through regular aerobic exercise that increases your heart rate to its Target Heart Rate Zone (THRZ) for 20 to 60 minutes, three to five times per week. Check with your physician about THRZ.
- Make the following dietary improvements:
  - Avoid high-cholesterol food sources such as egg yolks, liver, kidneys, and brains.
  - Follow American Heart Association guidelines. Reduce your fat intake to no more than 30 percent of your total calories. Make a special effort to reduce your consumption of saturated fats to no more than 10 percent of total fat calories.

    Saturated fats are usually of animal origin and have been found to actually raise blood cholesterol levels. Sour cream, lard, butter, solid (hydrogenated) vegetable shortening, and palm and coconut oils are examples of saturated fats.

    Plan instead to eat more whole grains, bran cereals (especially oat bran), fruits, vegetables, fish, poultry, and lean meats.

- Check your medications. A side effect of some medications is a lowered HDL level. If you are taking medications and have a low HDL level, check with your physician to see if your medication could be a factor.

DINING OUT TIPS

Do not be afraid to eat out. As long as you know your meal plan and choose foods wisely from the menu, dining should be enjoyable. Here are some tips that will help you:

1. Remember to eat only the portions permitted in your meal plan.
2. Consider the menu selection when choosing a restaurant.
3. If you are in a position where you feel you would offend your host if you do not sample a food, sample a small amount.
4. If you know your regular meal schedule will be delayed, eat lightly and "save" the remainder of your food allowance for dining out.
5. Do not hesitate to ask the waiter or waitress how a food is prepared (for example, breaded, fried, or added sugar).
6. If vegetables are cooked in fat, omit a fat exchange with the meal.
7. Ask for salad dressings and gravies to be served on the side.
8. Avoid fried, creamed, or au gratin entrées and vegetables.
9. Avoid sweet rolls, sweetened appetizers, and desserts. Avoid sweetened food items such as glazed or candied vegetables and entrées.
10. Avoid combination entrées if you are unsure how to count them in the exchange lists.

Bon Appétit!

Source: Memorial Medical Center of West Michigan

ETHNIC FOODS LIST

There are several ethnic recipes in this book. My ancestors came from Denmark, and my husband's ancestors are also Scandinavian. We have many friends from many cultures, and they have shared recipes with me through the years. I have modified them so they are low in sugar, cholesterol, and fat, and I have designated their origin.

Appetizers/Snacks

Italian Pita Squares
Onion Crisps, Norwegian Style
Popcorn, Southwest Spanish Style

Breads

Aebleskiver (Small Danish Pancake Balls)
Appelsin (Danish Orange Bread)

Soups

Cucumber Buttermilk Soup (Scandinavian)
Swedish Fruit Soup
Tortilla Soup (Mexican)

Salads

German Potato Salad

Meats and Casseroles

Frikadeller (Danish Meatballs)

Meatballs (Scandinavian Style)

Chicken Marengo (Italian)

Machaca (Mexican)

Beef and Pasta (Italian)

Sloppy Joe Pitas (Italian)

Burritos (Mexican)

Low-Calorie Lasagna (Italian)

Taco Casserole (Mexican)

Southwest Spanish Rice Casserole

Vegetables

German Style Sauerkraut

Sautéed Zucchini (Italian)

Desserts

Danish Apple Cake (Aeblekage)

Danish Rhubarb Dessert (Rabarbergrod)

Deep-Dish Pear Pie (Scandinavian)

Baked Custard (Scandinavian)

A SAMPLE WEEKLY LOG

This is an excerpt from my weekly log, but it is not meant to be used as a sample diet for a week. Rather, it is meant to show that diabetics do not have to eat "perfectly" at every meal. I chose this week because I ate out (and I ate leftovers) as most "normal" people do. This menu might make a certified diabetic educator cringe, but it did manage to keep my blood glucose readings under control, which is what diabetics try to achieve.

SUNDAY

Blood Glucose Readings		Exercise Record	
8:05 AM	113	Walking	2 miles
5:50 PM	97	Stairs	150 steps
		Exercise Bike	2 miles
		Stair-Stepper	¼ mile

Today's Menu

Breakfast: ½ cup Bran Flakes™ and ½ cup Special K™
½ cup 2% milk
1 medium banana; 10 red grapes

Lunch: Chicken salad—½ cup flaked chicken, 10 green grapes, and diet salad dressing
6 Club™ crackers
2 no-sugar almond cookies

Dinner: 4 oz. meat—beef and pork combination roast

½ cup mashed potatoes

½ cup broccoli casserole—broccoli, cheese, cream of mushroom soup, and baking mix

Salad—lettuce, tomato, and cucumber, plus 1 tablespoon low-calorie ranch dressing

Strawberry Shortcake—1 "Easy Sugar-Free Shortcake" (see recipe)

½ cup strawberries with no sugar added

2 teaspoons Lite Cool Whip™

PM Snack: ½ cup Weight Watchers Pecan Praline™ frozen dessert

MONDAY

Blood Glucose Readings

		Exercise Record	
7:55 AM	107	Walking	1½ miles
5:10 PM	98	Stairs	100 steps
		Exercise Bike	3 miles
		Stair-Stepper	none

Today's Menu

Breakfast: ½ cup Bran Flakes™ and ½ cup Special K™

½ cup 2% milk

1 medium banana; 10 red grapes

Lunch: 1 slice rye bread

2 oz. roast beef

10 Pringle's Lite Potato Chips™

2 teaspoons dip with sour cream and chopped beef

Dinner: 3 oz. meat—beef and pork combination roast

(leftovers) 1 tablespoon mashed potatoes

1 tablespoon broccoli casserole (same as Sunday)

Salad—lettuce, tomato, and cucumber, plus 1 table-
        spoon low-calorie ranch dressing
Strawberry Shortcake—1 "Easy Sugar-Free Short-
        cake" (see recipe)
½ cup strawberries with no sugar added
2 teaspoons Lite Cool Whip™
PM Snack: ½ cup strawberry frozen yogurt (no sugar added)

TUESDAY

Blood Glucose Readings		Exercise Record	
7:55 AM	107	Walking	2¼ miles
5:10 PM	98	Stairs	150 steps
		Exercise Bike	2 miles
		Stair-Stepper	¼ mile

Today's Menu

Breakfast:	½ cup Bran Flakes™ and ½ cup Special K™
	½ cup 2% milk
	1 medium banana; 10 red grapes
Lunch:	1 all-beef hot dog
	3 slices tomato
	10 Pringle's Lite Potato Chips™
	½ cup raspberry frozen dessert
Dinner:	3 oz. "Meatloaf" (see recipe)
	1 tablespoon mashed potatoes
	½ cup "Hash Brown Potato Casserole" (see recipe)
	½ cup green bean casserole—green beans, cream of mushroom soup, and canned onion rings
	Strawberry Shortcake—1 "Easy Sugar-Free Short-cake" (see recipe)
	½ cup strawberries with no sugar added
PM Snack:	½ cup raspberry frozen dessert

WEDNESDAY

Blood Glucose Readings		Exercise Record	
7:30 AM	94	Walking	1¼ miles
5:10 PM	94	Stairs	100 steps
		Exercise Bike	3 miles
		Stair-Stepper	none

Today's Menu

Breakfast: ½ cup Bran Flakes™ and ½ cup Special K™
½ cup 2% milk
1 medium banana; 10 red grapes

Lunch: Ate at mall food court—1 large piece of pizza with green pepper, pepperoni, and cheese
2 Estee™ peanut butter cookies
½ cup raspberry frozen dessert

Dinner: 2 "Meatballs (Scandinavian Style)" (see recipe)
½ cup mashed potatoes
½ cup steamed cauliflower
Green pepper slices and carrot sticks
2 Ritz™ crackers

PM Snack: ½ cup raspberry frozen dessert

THURSDAY

Blood Glucose Readings		Exercise Record	
7:30 AM	97	Walking	1½ miles
5:10 PM	97	Stairs	175 steps
		Exercise Bike	2 miles
		Stair-Stepper	½ mile

Today's Menu

Breakfast:	½ cup Bran Flakes™ and ½ cup Special K™
	½ cup 2% milk
	1 medium banana; 10 red grapes
Lunch:	1 slice rye bread
	2 oz. "Meatloaf" (see recipe)
	2 tablespoons green bean casserole (same as Tuesday)
	1 Weight Watchers Apple Crisp™ frozen dessert
Dinner:	1 bacon, lettuce, and tomato sandwich on 1 slice sourdough bread
	½ cup pistachio pudding salad—pudding, pine-apple, and Cool Whip™
	Sliced cucumber mandarin orange slices with Cool Whip™
	½ cup strawberry frozen yogurt
	2 no-sugar almond cookies
PM Snack:	½ cup Weight Watchers Pecan Praline™ frozen dessert

FRIDAY

Blood Glucose Readings		Exercise Record	
9:00 AM	91	Walking	1 mile
5:10 PM	99	Stairs	147 steps
		Exercise Bike	2½ miles
		Stair-Stepper	1 mile

Today's Menu

Breakfast:	½ cup Bran Flakes™ and ½ cup Special K™
	½ cup 2% milk
	1 medium banana; 10 red grapes

Lunch: 1 cup chicken noodle soup

5 Club™ crackers

1 Weight Watchers Apple Crisp™ frozen dessert

Dinner: 1 cup "Southwest Spanish Rice Casserole" (see recipe)

1 slice fresh tomato

Sliced cucumber

3 slices kiwi

10 red grapes

2 no-sugar almond cookies

½ cup vanilla frozen yogurt

PM Snack: 1 no-sugar almond cookie

SATURDAY

Blood Glucose Readings		Exercise Record	
8:30 AM	117	Walking	3¼ miles
6:10 PM	107	Stairs	129 steps
10:00 PM	104	Exercise Bike	1½ miles
		Stair-Stepper	none

Today's Menu

Breakfast: ½ cup Bran Flakes™ and ½ cup Special K™

½ cup 2% milk

1 medium banana; 10 red grapes

Lunch: Ate out: cup of cheese and broccoli soup

Tossed salad with croutons and "lite" ranch dressing

2 small pieces cornbread

1 small Breeze™ (Dairy Queen™ frozen yogurt dessert)

Dinner: 1 baked pork chop
2 tablespoons "Southwest Spanish Rice Casserole"
(see recipe)
Salad—lettuce, tomato, and green pepper, plus
1 tablespoon low-calorie ranch dressing
1 Weight Watchers™ strawberry dessert
PM Snack: 1 no-sugar almond cookie

SUNDAY

Blood Glucose Readings

7:05 AM   103

INDEX